# On Guard

Build Resilience — Boost Immunity — Beat Infection

**Functional Medicine helps you achieve a powerful immune system**

Gaynor J Greber

*For readers who are motivated by the healing power of nature and wish to promote their own health without the use of drugs.*

# About the Author

Gaynor Greber qualified with excellence from The Institute for Optimum Nutrition in London in 1993. As a Clinical Nutritionist and Functional Medicine Practitioner, she spent twenty-two years in private practice in the UK before moving to Switzerland.

She is currently a Senior Associate of the Royal Society of Medicine and a member of The Institute for Functional Medicine.

# Contents

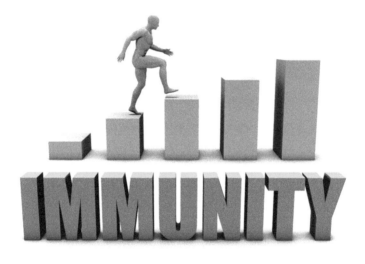

# INTRODUCTION

This book has been written with the lay person in mind. It does not attempt to impart complex medical knowledge using scientific language that may confuse readers, though certain terminology must be used in order to picture the scene.

It is intended as an easy to follow guide, which focuses on basic facts concerning immunity and valuable advice on how to enhance immune function by natural means.

It emphasises the need for a personal call to action, discusses the benefit of a healthy diet and lifestyle on immune function and offers drug-free options to help avoid or fight infection.

Regardless of the infective dangers of the world we live in – bugs literally everywhere: teeming on surfaces, inhabiting our bodies, food, water and air – one thing is certain, and should not be forgotten: our bodies do have an amazing protective defence system.

Our immune system provides us with the tools (white blood cells) to fight infection. A perfectly designed, complex, biological system with inbuilt warning signals, and multiple biochemical pathways that get activated at the first sign of danger.

We need to nourish this wonderful protective body system: not bypass it by reaching for a drug every time we feel unwell.

There are trillions of harmful micro-organisms in the environment, looking for the chance to inhabit your body – to snuggle inside a warm host with a plentiful supply of nourishment: a chance to flourish, thrive and multiply. There will always be the danger of new mutant strains developing in our ever-changing environment, some relatively benign and easy to recover from, and others that you certainly do not want to meet – more deadly. Not all microbes are bad though.

We carry around a huge community of micro-organisms within our bodies and cannot live without them. Our gut environment is teeming with bacteria, both beneficial and non-beneficial species, plus many viruses that can reside in the gut for years without causing symptoms.

It is the balance within the total microbiome (the sum of all the microbes on and in the human body) that counts, and this is kept in check by strong immune defences, and a healthy diet. Friendly bacteria residing in our gut help support immune function by protecting us against invading pathogens. They should represent a majority in your gut. Eat a poor diet and your beneficial friends will start to fade away, allowing the bad bugs to take over. This is bad news for the immune system; it could be in a constant state of 'overdrive' as it struggles to reduce infection.

Why? you might ask – if nature has provided us with this wonderful protective system, do we need to bother about further immune support? The answer is simple: the immune system can become damaged by faulty diet and unhealthy lifestyles; it can become damaged by the thousands of toxic chemicals floating round in our world.

Surviving and maintaining good health in an ever-increasing fast paced environment, dodging bugs and toxins, taxes reserves. The immune system can struggle under these conditions and fail to function optimally if care is not taken to live wisely and healthily. Every little effort counts.

Some people are more prone than others to picking up infection. Each person is biochemically unique. Immune function varies in every human being. There are many factors involved in the fight to keep fit: stress, environment, diet, lifestyle, genetic make-up – and at a deeper level – biochemical individuality; liver function, nutritional status, and detoxification capability.

People today are often in a general poor state of health; many overweight and unfit, with pot bellies and rolls of excess fat. These individuals may struggle to fight infection more than healthy individuals, when exposed to bugs. Recent studies have shown that people who are overweight are more likely to become seriously ill or have poor recovery rates.

Some people may, by nature, have an unhealthy mentality, 'Why bother with all this nonsense over diet and living a healthy lifestyle, let's just have fun, eat junk food and take a pill when all goes wrong'.

Sadly, for these individuals, the risk of picking up infections becomes higher.

How effectively you fight infection will depend on your general state of wellness and the efficiency of your immune system. The latter is ultimately dependent on the quality of your diet for nourishment, as you will read about later in this book.

It is not germs that determine the risk for disease; it is the power of your own body, the efficiency of your immune cells in resisting infection that limits the risk.

Viruses have been around since the beginning of time and have evolved with the human body, some remaining dormant, others invading resident gut bacteria or disrupting our own cellular DNA. Whether a body succumbs to infection is down to individual resilience.

Viruses interact with the host body, and in this way, are constantly evolving. New viruses are frequently being discovered – it is quite natural for them to inhabit the world and human bodies; this is how they survive, and they will keep mutating and spreading when conditions become favourable.

Now, more than ever, we need to get our body defences fortified: get our immune system functioning optimally.

Inappropriate use of antibiotics taken for minor infections will often suppress the ability of your immune army of white blood cells to control serious infection in the future. Antibiotics do not differentiate between good and bad bacteria: they will wipe out not only unhealthy bugs but a good percentage of friendly bugs.

Simple infections must be allowed to run their course. Boosting the body with active medicinal foods and potent herbal and nutritional remedies can offer the best immune support.

Individuals need to take responsibility for their own health.

Should serious infection develop, the person is then in a better state of resistance.

Some medics have started to question the wisdom of harsh drug treatments, unnecessary profitable surgical procedures, and overuse of diagnostic scans, that are thought to promote unhealthy cell changes.

They are beginning to understand that good health comes from within. Nutritional medicine is not taught in medical school, the focus is on the management of disease, not health.

Nutrients can be used as healing agents in the same manner as drugs, but without the side effects. Nutritional or Functional Medicine uses laboratory testing for assessing biochemical imbalance and dysfunction of body systems, applies corrective methods, using elements naturally present in the human body: a holistic natural approach to healing.

Many people are dependent on medication to see them through life: drug cocktails prescribed over years, sometimes by different health care providers, rarely given therapeutically, which is surely the object: but mostly prescribed for life. The original plot is then often lost as new symptoms develop from drug-related altered biochemistry.

Boosting immune function by natural means, a gentle stimulation – allows your immune system to function as nature intended.

Looking after your immune system by healthy living is your strongest protection against disease causing pathogens.

*The healthier you are – the lower the risk.*

This book is not intended to replace standard medical advice, but rather to supplement knowledge. It gives individuals options and choices for knowing how to build a strong immune system and improve resilience against infection and disease. If you have a diagnosed medical condition, you should seek professional advice when using information from this book.

'Disease is not an entity, but a fluctuating condition of the patient's body, a battle between the substance of disease and the natural healing powers of the body'

Hippocrates c 460 – 375 BC


'Look deep into nature and then you will understand everything better'

Albert Einstein 1879 – 1955

# OUR EVOLVING WORLD

Infectious diseases have always been around throughout history. Regardless of the current new deadly virus, today's pandemic is nothing new in historical terms. What is new, however, despite all modern scientific achievements, is society's inability to feel optimally protected against infection.

People are struggling to keep fit and well. There is panic as people realise, they may be more vulnerable than they thought.

What has gone wrong?

In medieval times, poverty and disease in the lower strata of society was rife, and effective medicine or drug development just a dream away. People relied on cures from nature.

Living conditions for both well-off and poor households were unsanitary and filthy. Garbage, animal remains, human waste – all ended up in rivers, city drains, garden soil, or simply lying where it was originally thrown – a breeding ground for pests and disease. Under these conditions, people succumbed easily to sickness and poor health. They were more prone to getting infections and less able to fight them. The poor suffered from poverty and malnourishment and they had a shorter lifespan.

People feasted largely on animal products, and what was available from the garden, often contaminated with bacteria. There was no concept of safe food preservation, only the valuable knowledge of protective herbs and plants, and even this knowledge did not include accurate dosing or correct choice, as science was in its infancy concerning the recognition of individual properties contained in each herb.

It was a little hit and miss: but it was all they had.

Much medical treatment was gathered from 'old wives' tales' or hearsay. There was a good deal of 'trial and error,' but nevertheless with the benefit of today's discoveries, we can see that ancient society was certainly on the right route.

Similar conclusions were reached in different countries, different faiths, and beliefs, by different means – nature has certainly been reaped over millennium for the benefit of mankind. Old scripts, full of herbal wisdom and knowledge, have in modern times been proven correct in content.

The potential healing power of medicinal plants, and essential wisdom from learned individuals, grew over years, was added to, and improved upon. Monks and scribes involved in the study of plant life analysed, to the best of their ability, the properties in herbs, and pondered appropriate medical applications.

This knowledge, passed down through the ages, is as valuable today as it was then.

The benefit of a healthy diet and effective healing knowledge was unknown of course, apart from wise comments from ancient philosophers, such as Hippocrates, who preached the term: 'Help the sick, and do no harm', and the early theories of medicinal alchemy from Paracelsus in the sixteenth century, writing prolifically about the magical properties of herbs and the value of observation. He wrote that harmony between nature and humans and a correct balance of minerals in the body: were pre-requisites for good health.

Diets for the well off in medieval times was rich, and gout was common. People ate multiple meat, fish and fowl courses, all washed down with wine or beer as water was regarded as unclean. Immense amounts of animal fat, and later sugar and refined grains – unhealthy carbohydrates – were added to the mix.

The only dietary benefit for society in those days, compared to today, was the lack of processed food and the thousands of artificial chemicals used in our food industry.

## LONGER LIFESPAN – SICKER SOCIETY

Our diet today may not be rich and gluttonous, but the intake of calories is often far in excess of the body's requirements and the quality of the calories eaten often leaves much to be desired. The danger and risk of becoming sick and ill exists in other forms.

Public health figures make alarming reading today; degenerative conditions, obesity, diabetes, auto-immune disease: all on the increase. General sub-optimal health and poor immunity add to the picture: life has swung far to the opposite side of the pendulum.

People in the Western world are not suffering from poverty, but they *are* suffering from an excess of processed foods, deficient in nutrients, unhealthy and chemically laden.

Tempting to look at: but risky to eat – if you have health in mind.

Most people would be shocked to learn that the food they put in their bodies may be harming them. Shocked if they read reports on intensive farming procedures, pesticide residues, chemical additives, the toxic rubbish one is expected to ingest with food.

A gradual slide into ill health, when the body's reserves get depleted and the immune system fails to protect you from infection and disease – doesn't happen overnight. It takes time and sometimes years of bad habits before your body fails to renew body tissues and repair itself correctly.

It can take years for the first symptoms of poor health to appear.

Listening to your body pays dividends. The body has strong built-in mechanisms for long-term recovery, providing it receives the right conditions and nutritious fuel (nutrients) to make these changes. Far better to have foresight and awareness of the cause and effect of poor health than suffer and repair the damage.

We can protect ourselves from infectious diseases by strengthening our defences, nourishing our bodies and maintaining a strong immune system.

The good thing about the human body is that it sends out signals when all is not well. You do have many warning signs along life's path that give you time for altering course; ignoring them of course is not the wisest thing to do.

Your one and only body relies on you to protect it; there is no replacement round the corner.

Many young people consider it normal to race around like there is no tomorrow, cramming in as much hectic sociable living hours as possible – enjoying a fast pace of life that generally stresses their body to the limit.

Living in a world surrounded by man-made electromagnetic fields doesn't help either: the body's own electrical field is being constantly challenged and disturbed. Most humans are linked to cell tower connections or exposed to electromagnetic fields for every action of every day; and a future with satellite tower connections beamed direct to your phone is looming.

# On Guard

There is not a lot to be done about modern technology; this is developing at a rate far beyond what our bodies can cope with – only time will tell how damaging this may be. People love their gadgets; health, documented studies on cellular damage from man-made electromagnetic fields, is not up for discussion: that would entail curbing lifestyle.

New gadgets increase steadily year by year, and there is no guarantee that the body possesses unlimited compensation mechanisms to counterbalance these biological effects.

Personal choice on exposure limitation is your only protection against environmental pollutants.

We will never fully conquer the bugs that thrive in our world, because they are opportunists who prey on vulnerable weak individuals or communities with poor living standards.

We can, however, take action to protect ourselves with potent agents from nature, as the advice in this book emphasises.

Potentially deadly microbes, strains of bacteria, viruses, parasites and fungi that are resistant to drugs have developed over time and are now a threat to society. They enter your body through the mouth, nose or from open injuries.

Once established, a weakened body will struggle to fight against these pathogens (disease causing bugs) which reproduce rapidly in the human body. They attack and destroy cells: secreting noxious toxins into your bloodstream.

It sounds a sinister and alarming picture, and it is, but there is a lot you can do to be on guard and mount a counter attack.

It is well worth remembering you are not a defenceless individual, who needs to rely on some magic drug that comes your way. Your body has the means to fight infection and build a strong defence, even against new strains of deadly bacteria or viruses.

What's more: it is never too late. Your body is self-healing, it has in-built powers of recovery for rejuvenating weak or infected cells – you just need to be aware that the basic tools you need are powerful nutrients from your diet and medicinal support from herbs.

Following universally advised measures to avoid transmission of these potentially deadly germs is vital. It would also be wise to take a range of protective nutrients and herbal products.

This information is covered extensively later on in this book.

If you think you have been infected and before you may start to feel unwell, you can launch your arsenal of super foods and potent infection-fighting natural agents. You will instantly be strengthening your defences and hopefully avoiding illness.

Should you need urgent medical care, or hospitalisation, you will respond more favourably to drug treatment as your body will be in a better state of general health.

## FACTORS INFLUENCING IMMUNITY

### Biochemical individuality

Even in families, there is no one exactly like yourself.

Resistance to disease can be only partially inherited, the rest is in your hands; how you choose to live, how well you nourish your body, determines how your inherited genes behave.

The actual expression of inherited genes – how well your body protects you – is dependent upon your personal metabolic make-up, nutritional balance, dietary choices, lifestyle, environmental conditions, stress levels, and exposure to toxins.

It is no good looking – as the saying goes – 'at Joe Bloggs, down the street,' he does not have your genes: your biological make-up.

And if Grandad died at the ripe old age of ninety and chain smoked all his life. He was just lucky; one out of fifty just might survive that long. You may not if you have the same habit.

Life is not a game of 'Russian Roulette' – and it's really the quality of life that counts. Could Grandad have climbed hills without being short of breath? Did he need medication, and limitation on activities that stressed the heart?

If Granny kept fit throughout her life, eating well and following a healthy lifestyle, and you choose to smoke, drink, eat unhealthily, party late, avoid exercise and generally abuse your body, you can't rely on her inherited genes to keep you fit.

In this over populated, under nourished – as far as nutrients are concerned – world around us, it is even harder to keep truly healthy, surrounded as we are by mountains of tantalising unhealthy goodies.

Years ago, there was little choice in food – what was given on the plate, was what was available. There were no options to offer children or adults. There were no supermarkets to attract you to junk food. Fewer calories, basic choice, but unadulterated unprocessed food: generally rich in nutrients.

Modern intensive agricultural practices have given more choice but at the expense of health.

There has been a steady reduction in food quality since supermarkets emerged.

Children are asked today what they would like for meals. Unable to verbalise 'Healthy food please!' they quite naturally go for the advertised junk food. and end up having an unhealthy diet and a bad habit for life.

Allowing children to choose meals themselves, at the expense of teaching them healthy dietary habits, is a recipe for disaster.

A better option is to choose a selection of healthy nutritional options – then give them a choice.

There are many healthy treats available and numerous sugar-free recipe books. Learning nutrition at a young age means a healthier body in old age.

Every human being responds differently, when exposed to environmental pollutants in the environment. The type of response is dependent on the health of your liver.

## Toxins

Food additives (there are over 80,000 chemicals used today in the food industry) can overload this organ, which metabolises and excretes toxins. Synthetic chemicals have no place in the human body; they simply benefit the food industry in very cheaply enhancing flavour and building profit by prolonging shelf life.

You may have a wonderful cleaning up system in your liver, but there is a limit to the rubbish you can take in. Pushing detoxification pathways beyond capacity, by eating processed food, is not giving your body an easy ride.

The lower the toxin load: the healthier the immune system.

There will always be different risks of disease faced by mankind, due to location, genetic make-up, environment, lifestyle, and diet.

## A Healthy Gut

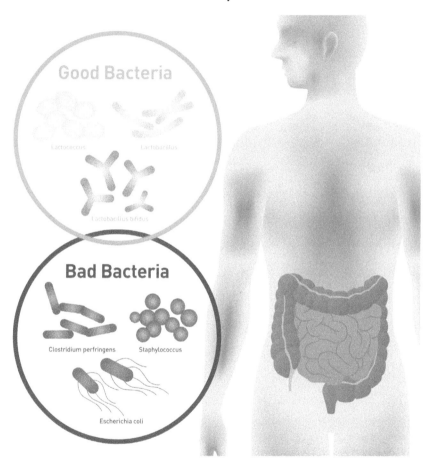

Improved Immunity

The answer, in general terms, involves making your body stronger, healthier, and hardy enough to resist disease.

We do have choices: which foods to avoid, what lifestyle to lead. There is no reason to be unhealthy.

## Intestinal health

*Approximately one in four persons suffers from digestive complaints.*

Having healthy digestion and well-functioning bowels supports good immunity and helps keep you fighting fit. An enormous community of organisms, known as the microbiome, lives inside your gut.

Having a healthy microbiome is probably the most important thing you can do to enhance immunity. From birth on, good immunity is initially established by breast feeding, and further supported by healthy eating habits.

For every cell in your body there are at least ten-fold numbers of microbes snuggled down, living happily within you. Nature has designed our bodies for good and bad bacteria to co-exist in a balanced fashion.

Health problems only loom when undesirable microbes take over the show, and beneficial organisms that work to keep the body healthy struggle to survive.

These trillions of live micro-organisms residing in our gut weigh approximately 3-5 lbs, with most of this mass in good health, favouring beneficial species of bacteria.

The immune system is distributed throughout your entire body, but approximately 70% of your immune cells live in your intestinal tract. So, keeping your gut healthy keeps your immune system in good order.

Keeping hydrated will also enable your immune cells to function well. Most people with digestive problems have an imbalance in gut organisms and may suffer from bacterial overgrowth – a condition called dysbiosis. Unless these gut problems are resolved, it can damage immune function.

After digestion of food, the absorption of nutrients takes place through the gut lining – a tight barrier in the small intestine. If this tight junction becomes more permeable from dysbiosis (microbial imbalance) it can cause a leaky gut, allowing toxins to 'leak' into the bloodstream, activate the immune system, and cause allergic reactions.

A leaky gut can challenge the immune system and put it in attack mode. It can also lead to auto-immune disorders, where the body attacks its own cells, causing dysfunctional body systems.

Most people with poor immunity have a disturbed, less than healthy bowel flora or internal gut environment. Healthy levels of beneficial bacteria keep pathogenic bacteria in check, fight infection and have many other important roles: helping detoxification, sanitising your bowels, synthesizing B vitamins, and producing vitamin K.

Beneficial Lactobacilli bacteria live in your small intestine and help fight infection by producing antibacterial substances: lactic acid that helps destroy pathogens. The Bifidobacterium species live in your large bowel and help prevent infection by producing acetic acid and lactic acid, natural antibiotics that fight off unhealthy invaders.

Both species can be found in quality live yoghurts.

Damaged Gut Lining

# Leaky gut syndrome

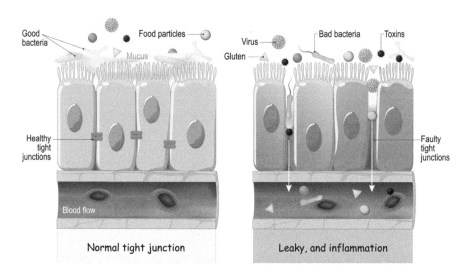

Suppresses Immunity

You can appreciate how important it is to keep your gut in good health. My book 'Chronic Digestive Disorders' covers this subject in some detail and shows you how to reverse symptoms and regain health.

Restoring healthy bacterial balance in the gut will improve your immune function. The whole ecosystem is extraordinarily complex; this is the one area that only you can influence.

Having a healthy gut environment is vital in helping to protect your body against disease, this is one area where you can have control through sensible dietary choice. Studies have shown that the microbiome influences and helps modulate the immune response.

A substantial percentage of immune system cells called 'Peyer's patches' are in the intestinal tract, and it is this close relationship between gut and immune function, which necessitates the need for a healthy bacterial balance which favours friendly microbes.

Beneficial bacteria have been shown to communicate with both the innate and adaptive immune branches, ensuring the correct response against pathogen attack. They form a protective barrier to deter bugs and toxins from attaching to gut cells.

Prebiotics in plant food (non-digestible fibre) stimulate growth of beneficial Bifidobacterium and Lactobacillus species in the gastrointestinal tract using a process of fermentation. As friendly gut bacteria ferment fibre from plant food in the colon, short chain fatty acids are produced, which benefit gut and immune health by providing energy and nutrients.

Chemicals and various acids in fermented foods also play a valuable part in keeping bugs at bay and helping to prevent infection.

To improve strength and efficiency of your immune function, a varied intake of the following foods should be eaten to increase growth of beneficial bacteria:

**Prebiotic foods include – onions, garlic, leeks, artichokes, bananas, apples, chicory root, berries, grains and other fibre rich fruit and vegetables.**

**Probiotic fermented foods – yoghurt, kefir, kimchi, pickles, sauerkraut, miso, tempeh, cheese and sourdough.**

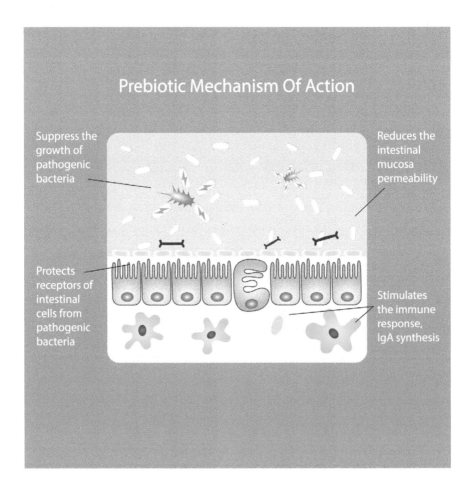

# PART ONE
# THE NATURE OF BUGS

## Bacteria

These are amongst the smallest single cell organisms. They live just about everywhere: in soil, water, airborne, in and on all living beings. Their structure looks like small rods and dots under the microscope.

Basic good hygiene will limit the rate of bacterial infections picked up by humans. Some bacteria, though, can cause serious disease. They replicate rapidly under favourable conditions: warmth and nourishment.

Sugar in any form is a desirable bacterial food, so addressing this one fact alone can limit the spread within the body.

Bacterial infections can produce a stimulatory effect in the body which speeds up metabolic function; this can result in chills or fever.

Bacteria develop a protective mechanism – a slimy glue-like substance – a mantle, called a *Biofilm* which wraps around their structure, making destruction difficult. The trick for helping to get rid of bacterial infections is to is to make living conditions for pathogens undesirable.

A sugar-free diet for instance, using antimicrobial herbs, garlic, pepper, juniper and strong spices in food. Taking vitamin C rich foods, and at least 1,000mg of vitamin C daily. Having anti-microbial, antioxidant, anti-inflammatory properties, this vitamin works wonders when taken regularly.

Saturating body tissues protects cells and fights infection.

Health-giving nutrients and disease fighting herbs, constantly flooding the body, support your immune army.

You must eat anyway, so why not make your meals packed full of antioxidant, antimicrobial food chemicals that keep your internal body clean and healthy, Rather like hoovering up and having a regular spring-clean internally.

If you have healthy digestion and fully digest your food, this ensures there is no partially digested debris left in the gut, for pathogenic bacteria to survive on.

## Viruses

These organisms are even smaller than bacteria and come in different shapes that can only be identified microscopically. Despite their size, viruses can cause a huge amount of damage to your body. They do not live off the host body, and they do not replicate in the same fashion as bacteria.

The cell structure is simple: a coil of genes wrapped up in protein. The protein contains projections that can hook onto human or animal cells, increasing hold and replication. Viruses can thrive for years in your gut without causing symptoms, then, when defences are low – when you are rundown or stressed – they can activate and cause illness.

They can only survive inside cells of living organisms if your immunity is under-functioning. If your immune defences are strong, you are less likely to succumb to viral infection, as viruses are self-limiting, which means they can be controlled by a well-functioning immune system.

Viruses can only survive outside a body for a short period of time. Inside your body they latch onto your cells and use the contents to reproduce new versions of themselves, killing the cell in the process. The process is repetitious: different kinds of viruses can attack different cells anywhere in your body.

Viruses and bacteria treat the body like a breeding ground if allowed, but in efficient immune controlled healthy bodies their presence can also help build immunity.

## Parasites

These are multi celled organisms that live in another organism and depend on it for survival. Depending on the sort of diet you eat, they can either thrive or die. As blood suckers, they can live off the host quite adequately. This is an essential part of their survival tactic. Parasites are adapted to live in certain host environments and can cause untold damage in the human body.

A good thing to know is that parasites can be destroyed very efficiently by antimicrobial agents in certain herbs and food plants. Examples of parasites are worms, mites, lice, fleas, amoebas and tape worms. Eating unclean food abroad, handling animals and having poor hygiene can increase risk of infection.

## Fungi

Fungi are yeast microorganisms that produce spores and get nourished by the nutrient uptake in living hosts.

Fungal overgrowth can be localised in the human body or spread systemically throughout the body by long filaments to any organ – this is called a mycelial form. Certain conditions favour fungal overgrowth: warmth and especially moist areas of your body.

Factors such as a diet high in refined carbohydrates, sugar or alcohol intake feed yeast – as anyone knows, if they make homemade alcohol.

Antibiotic use can also promote fungal overgrowth. Living in old houses with poor damp proofing, or wet environments with musty conditions, can put you at greater risk for picking up fungal infections.

## Symptoms associated with infection of *Candida albicans* – a type of fungal overgrowth that thrives on sugar:

- IBS – digestive complaints, bloating, flatulence, loose stools
- Fatigue and low energy levels
- Cystitis, thrush, prostatitis, vaginitis, PMS, endometriosis
- Skin rashes, itching, re-occurrent infections
- Sugar cravings, 'foggy' brain, depression, anxiety, poor concentration
- Inability to lose weight

## Common signs of fungal overgrowth:

- Looking puffy under the eyes, being overweight with excess rings of fat around the middle.
- Dark lines under the eyes, with dull, poor skin quality.
- Feeling 'achy' all over.
- Always craving carbohydrates.

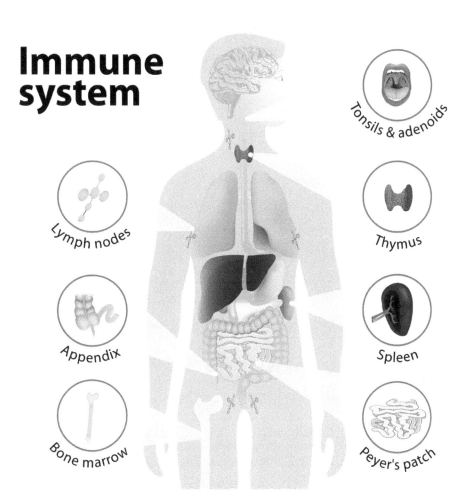

# THE IMMUNE SYSTEM

The main organs of the immune system are the tonsils, lymph nodes, spleen, bone marrow and thymus. In these organs the immune cells fight off infection.

Fighting disease is the job of your white blood cells – the immune 'army'. These are the main defenders within the immune system, and they are constantly on alert for attack, ready to protect your body.

This attack can be in the form of pathogens: bacteria, viruses, fungi or parasites or foreign material that enters the body in the form of damaging chemicals or toxins.

Even natural plant-based chemicals, naturally produced by food to protect themselves from attack, can activate the immune system and prompt an allergic reaction. In all instances the body is made aware of the invasion and takes appropriate action.

The immune function, a complicated network, is divided into innate (natural immunity) and acquired (adaptive immunity) responses.

## The Innate Immune System

The natural, first line of response takes place immediately when the body is exposed to an invader or pathogen. Alarm bells ring as a chemical substance on a pathogen – a surface protein, called an antigen, activates the immune system. This immune warning is designed to prevent the movement and spread of the invader throughout the body.

This first response is aided by a series of barriers in the body that keep damaging invaders from entering the body:

- The skin
- Mucous membranes
- Hairs, tears, saliva, urine
- The acid-alkaline balance on skin
- Sebum: the oily substance secreted by skin
- The sweat glands
- Acidic gastric juices

As an invader attacks, an immune memory cell triggers an alert for the second phase: the adaptive immune system to launch a defence counter attack.

A wonderfully complex army of cells that all work together to help keep you safe and healthy.

## The Adaptive Immune System

This system involves the production of specialised white blood cells to fight infection:

- T cells – which regulate the entire immune response
- B cells – which secrete antibodies
- Antibodies – which neutralize foreign material

There are many types of white blood cells, which all contribute to immune defence: memory cells, natural killer cells, messenger cells, neutrophils, eosinophils, basophils, monocytes, macrophage, and lymphocytes.

# CELL-MEDIATED IMMUNE RESPONSE

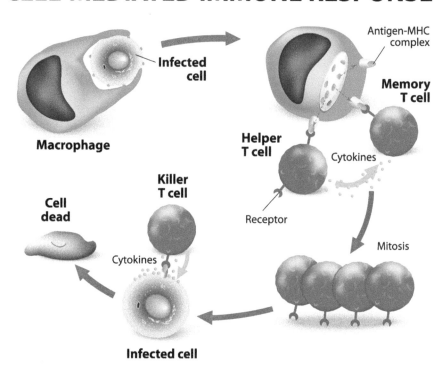

## Phagocytes

These specialised cells are key players. Produced by macrophages, they destroy germs by enveloping and absorbing them. They can reach germs in unusual places, by changing shape and wriggling through blood capillaries.

When you see inflammation (histamine) at an injury site, this is a sign of phagocyte activity. The body increases metabolism and switches on the heating, which quickly brings white blood cells into action.

It is therefore not a good thing to reduce a temperature, unless it rises dangerously. The extra heat is there to fight pathogens. Inflammation confines the microbes and destroys them, then repairs the tissue: the heat speeds up body reactions that help repair.

## Antibodies

Antibodies are produced by B cells of the adaptive immune system in response to invasion. They are adapted to combine specifically with different shapes and sizes of antigens and then circulate throughout the body destroying the culprits.

They cause destruction of germs by attacking the antigen, a protein on its surface, killing the germ in the process.

Some antibodies make the germs 'burst' so that the phagocytes can come along and finish them off. A wonderfully intricate system of patrol, invasion and destruction.

**There are five classes of antibodies. The Ig stands for Immunoglobulins – a type of protein.**

Ig A, G, E, D and M antibodies all have specific functions to help you fight infection.

## IgA

Is the most common antibody and is a potent defence substance. It is secreted on all mucosal surfaces of your body. It can be found in the lining of your gut and lungs and is the first line of defence against foreign invaders: viruses, bacteria, fungi or parasites.

It acts by neutralizing the foreign body and preventing attachment to cell walls, so it is an unbelievably valuable antibody.

Deficiency of IgA showing up on a blood or stool test is an overall marker of poor immunity.

## IgG

Is an antibody found in blood and body fluids; it protects you against viral and bacterial attack but is also involved in allergic reactions of a delayed nature, such as food intolerance. The immune reaction can take place hours or days after ingesting an offending food that has caused rejection in the body.

## IgM

This antibody is found in blood and lymph fluid. This is the first antibody produced in the various stages of fighting infection.

## IgD

Is an antibody found in small amounts in the body. It has a minor function in helping to signal B cell activity.

## IgE

This antibody is involved in hypersensitivity, an immediate allergic reaction to food antigens, or environmental substances, such as pollen, animal hair or chemical toxins. These are mostly genetically inherited reactions of a severe nature, which can be present lifelong. Called atopic allergies, they can provoke serious life-threatening anaphylactic shock.

Great care is needed to avoid the suspected antigen.

## Immune checklist

## Do you:

- **Pick up infections easily?**
- **Visit the doctor frequently for minor complaints?**
- **Have trouble shaking off coughs and colds?**
- **Take a long time to recover from illness?**
- **Often feel 'under the weather,' or 'out of sorts'?**
- **Suffer from side-effects of long-term medication?**

## Immunity and body chemistry

Various mineral imbalances can lead to metabolic and immune dysfunction.

Warning signs such as these above should prompt you to look closely at your dietary and lifestyle habits.

If you need help, seek the advice of a Nutritional Therapist or Functional Medicine practitioner. They are trained to assess and treat biochemical imbalance.

They may suggest a range of tests, including blood, stool, urine or hair mineral analysis, to identify possible nutritional deficiencies, maldigestion, malabsorption, toxic overload or hormonal imbalance – all factors relating to poorly functioning body systems.

## Hair Mineral Analysis

Hair is a biological sample that reflects the deposition and mineral storage in your body tissues over a period of months. Hair tissue analysis can therefore be especially useful in providing a long-term record of normal or abnormal metabolism.

It is, however, important to use a reputable laboratory for testing procedures.

The body's sensitive mineral balance can influence a person's risk factors for picking up bacterial or viral infections.

Zinc, iron and copper ratios are important factors linked to immune efficiency.

People with chronic infections have been shown to have a high tissue iron to copper ratio; this tissue level is opposite to that seen in blood. Blood circulates, mineral deposits in tissues show storage levels.

During infection, bacteria takes iron from the blood in order to proliferate, and at the same time the body uses stored copper to help fight the infection.

Mineral balance is quite a complicated issue and is not something the average person can concern themselves with. I mention a few facts here that may be useful if you are considering seeing a practitioner.

Low copper levels can be seen in people with chronic bacterial infections; high copper levels are associated with a predisposition to recurring viral or fungal infections. Taking synthetic hormones is often one of the causes of developing high tissue copper, as copper is intricately linked to fluctuating oestrogen levels.

Nutrients such as vitamin A, zinc and vitamin C can be considered anti-viral as they reduce retention of copper and help keep copper tissue levels in balance.

Impaired immune function can also be indicated on hair mineral analysis when abnormal sodium and potassium ratios are seen. This affects the oxidation rate: the rate we burn (digest) food for energy. The immune system depends on adequate biochemical energy from the digestion of food.

**Factors that inhibit healthy immune function:**

- **Imbalanced diet, unhealthy dietary choices, alcohol, smoking**
- **Nutritional deficiencies, lack of exercise**
- **Medications, lack of sleep, chronic stress**
- **Excessive exposure to environmental and dietary toxins, man-made magnetic fields**
- **Gut dysbiosis – imbalance of micro-organisms in the intestinal tract**
- **Poor detoxification pathways and liver function**

## THE LYMPHATIC SYSTEM

The Lymphatic system consists of a fluid called lymph, which contains up to 90% water. This fluid collects drainage from all body systems: toxins, chemical garbage from food metabolism and dead pathogens. The lymph is then transported throughout parts of the immune system for excretion.

It works as an information and transportation network, filtering, hoovering up and transporting foreign substances out of the body. We have an effective immune system that destroys pathogens, and we need an effective lymph system to transport the waste out of the body: both systems have vital roles.

Organs in the lymphatic system consist of the tonsils, lymph nodes, spleen and thymus gland. The lymphatic tissue can be viewed as a defence mechanism, protecting the body from foreign microbial debris and other damaging substances.

Your tonsils produce lymphocytes and antibodies; your spleen destroys harmful bacteria and helps antibody production; and your thymus gland produces T cells that focus on destroying microbes.

Exercise is not only healthy: it also increases lymph flow. Toxins and wastes are then shifted along more readily to excretion sites. It becomes, however, less efficient if you become dehydrated.

So, every reason to get active if you want better immunity. If your body becomes sluggish, and your internal spring-cleaning system struggles, you run the risk of re-cycling dead pathogens instead of excreting them, making yourself unwell in the process.

Exercise not only boosts the metabolic rate; it can benefit every system in the body. As you move waste out of the body, production of antibodies increases, phagocytosis improves and so does your overall immunity and feeling of wellbeing.

There are natural antimicrobial substances secreted by the body when it is in good health: Interferon, Complement and Properdin.

These substances help protect the body from infection. Interferon specifically helps defend your body against viral infection.

## Vaccines

It is reported that many people are waiting for the ultimate COVID-19 vaccine that will save us all.

Most vaccines contain adjuvants – chemicals that provoke artificial immune stimulation and responses. People with weak liver detoxification pathways can fail to metabolise these body damaging chemicals efficiently, potentially causing unwanted side-effects.

Vaccines cause accelerated antibody production, by alerting the immune system to action.

They can overwhelm weak immune systems – by introducing foreign material direct into the blood stream. They are obviously designed to do just this – to provoke an immune response, but there is risk attached.

This is not how immunisation occurs naturally. The human body is designed to produce antibodies in response to infection without being artificially challenged by pharmaceuticals. Bypassing our natural immune response or prompting it to overreact is not a healthy option.

Years ago, weak vaccines were used, made from particles of pathogen that had been inactivated by heat, radiation or chemicals, such as formaldehyde.

Today vaccines can be synthesized or made by using modified viral material. They may still contain formaldehyde, antibiotics, egg protein, squalene or undesirable toxic metals to maximise immune response.

Methods of cultivation include culturing in chick embryos. The cultures are supposed to be so dilute that disease cannot be caused but these vaccines may, if live, on occasion revert to an active form that can cause disease.

Cellular structure and biochemistry constantly change throughout life; long-term safety of foreign material in a human body cannot be guaranteed.

The oral polio vaccine given to children in the 1950s was contaminated with a cancer-causing virus SV-40. Incidence of stomach cancer has been found in people from this generation. Analysis of tumour material pointed to a causal link with these contaminated batches.

I advise readers to read Lynne McTaggart's book on vaccines, listed in the Bibliography section. Also, her excellent magazine *What Doctors Don't Tell You*.

If you have faith and believe the medical field always works in your favour, your eyes will be opened.

## A chemical mix

Our body consists totally of chemical substances. Carbohydrates, fat, protein, salt and water.

We are approximately 18% protein, 10% fat, 5% carbohydrate, 2% other organic or inorganic substances, and 65% water.

These are the macro elements; the micro elements are the nutrients – vitamins and minerals.

All these substances come from our diet.

Our diet counts – we are, as they say – what we eat.

Poor health doesn't come from a deficiency of drugs but can come from a deficiency of nutrients – the raw materials that make up the human body.

# IMMUNE SYSTEM STRESSORS

## Alcohol

Alcohol has no nutritional value, apart from an antioxidant effect from the grapes in wine, and this effect is quickly negated by the damaging effect of alcohol itself.

Contrary to belief, certainly in those who like a regular tipple or two, alcohol *is* a stressor on body systems.

To name a few effects: it dehydrates, numbs the brain, reduces thought processes, and compromises judgement. And if this was not enough, it reduces nutrient stores.

The liver has the job of metabolising and eliminating alcohol out of your body, and valuable nutrients from your diet are used for this process: nutrients that could be put to better use.

Vitamins A, C, B complex, zinc, and magnesium, can quickly become depleted, if you are a regular or binge drinker.

Alcohol can also interfere with the process of digestion. It provides only empty calories, and, as an acidic substance, can cause digestive problems.

This is not to say, you should forgo the pleasure of all social drinking, but it should be taken in moderation.

However, if you are prone to picking up infections, have digestive problems or suffer with ill health, then alcohol should be avoided.

## Coffee

Coffee not only contains caffeine, a major stimulant, but two other stimulating substances: theobromine and theophylline. With regular intake, the constant stimulating effects on the hormonal system can disrupt blood sugar levels and suppress your immune function.

It is addictive, can cause sleepless nights, increase nervous tension, and stop you from relaxing.

Occasional intake of mild coffee will not harm, but regular intake of strong coffee will impact hormonal health.

It is important to remember that both tea and coffee de-hydrate the body, and you need water for your immune and lymphatic systems to function well.

## Sugar

This substance is the cause of many degenerative diseases. It is acidic forming and destructive in the human body: a nutrient robber. Hidden in many foods as a cheap taste enhancer, it has no value as food.

You can only appreciate the damage it causes and understand how it can make you feel unwell or cause gut problems when you avoid it completely.

Sugar can lead to numerous health problems. Blood sugar imbalance, sugar cravings, fungal overgrowth, diabetes, digestive complaints, bowel disorders, sleeplessness, anxiety, allergies, inflammation, hyperactivity, infections and cardiovascular disease.

Pathogens love sugar! White blood cell performance can be reduced for hours after the intake of just a few teaspoons of sugar. This is bad news for people trying to keep a healthy immune system.

It is often the reason why some people who have a high sugar intake are more prone to picking up infections.

## Medication

Immune cells are dependent on the action of friendly bacteria, so any medication can have a depressed effect on your gut immunity, as medication alters the balance of microbes. Particularly – non-steroidal anti-inflammatory drugs, corticosteroids, synthetic hormones and antibiotics.

For the body to metabolise and excrete pharmaceutical drugs, it needs a plentiful supply of nutrients, and as already mentioned, this can lead to dietary deficiencies.

Seeking natural alternative treatment for chronic health conditions can protect your immune system.

## Processed food

Processing food causes a high percentage of nutrients to be lost. Sometimes up to 70% of minerals and trace elements are lost in the processing of white flour, for instance. As your cell structures and body tissues are made from protein, fat and minerals, and cells only have a certain lifespan, you need to keep a regular flow of nutrients and sufficient reserves for replenishment.

Not only does the diet need to contain these essential nutrients, but the body also needs to digest and absorb them efficiently for utilisation in the cells.

We cannot use food in the form it is eaten in. Enzymes must digest your meals into a form that is ready for absorption.

If your intestinal tract is working well (you have no digestive complaints), then efficient digestion and absorption should take place.

Processed food is manipulated by man to produce a long shelf life, is low in essential nutrients, high in fat, salt and sugar, and laden with artificial additives.

This is not to say quick meals should be banished from your life for ever; rather, use them judiciously, for the times when you are too tired or too busy to cook.

Be careful in choice – read labels, choose organic, additive-free food where possible as the nutrient content is higher.

## Stress

The human body cannot function without some stress. It is part of normal metabolic function, and we produce hormones to manage it.

When stress gets out of control, however, and becomes chronic – *this* is when it can impact the immune system.

It is a well-recognised fact, that unresolved stress can make you more susceptible to infection. Your requirement for anti-stress nutrients goes up when the body is under pressure. Depletion of anti-stress nutrients, such as B vitamins, vitamin C, magnesium, and zinc are some of the same nutrients you need for healthy immunity.

## Dehydration

Being well hydrated helps absorption processes and brings nutrients to the cells, aids detoxification processes, lymphatic drainage and excretion of toxins.

Regularly hydrating your body helps all the metabolic processes.

The Stress Cycle

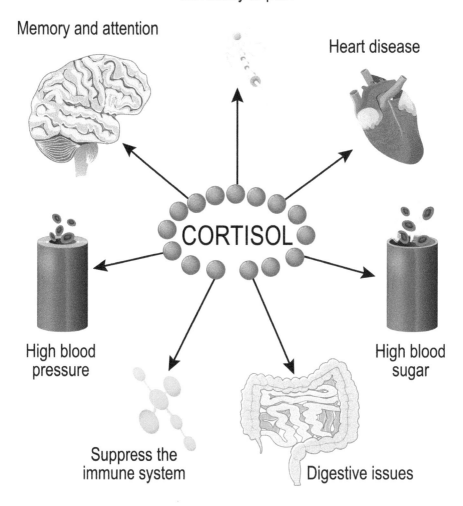

Effects of Excess Cortisol

Sleep apnoea and snoring are distinct signs of dehydration. Taking a final drink of water before bedtime will help flush out toxins overnight.

If you think this will increase night time toilet trips, don't worry; you will find the body adjusts in time.

A small amount of pure apple juice, which contains potassium, added to the water will ensure a slower kidney filtration rate.

From snoring like a traction engine to sleeping like a babe – hydrating all day and drinking last thing at night works wonders.

This does not mean drinking gallons to saturate the body, as this can have the opposite effect: flushing out vital nutrients.

Just drink enough to keep all body tissues bathed in fluid, to improve body function, digestion, absorption and utilisation of nutrients in your cells.

You may ask, 'How will I know when I have reached this stage?' This is hard to identify, but dehydration sets in an hour or so before the thirst sensation appears.

Signs of dehydration, apart from snoring, can include – headaches, lack of concentration, a 'fuzzy' head, panic attacks, hyperventilation and anxiety.

Observe your body messages, drink a glass of water every two hours and you will find your own balance.

You will also be able to think more clearly, have a better level of concentration and the added benefit of healthy skin and lubricated joints.

## Lack of exercise and fresh air

Exercise, not intense endurance but regular aerobic exercise, improves immune function. Exercising in gyms and indoor spaces tones the body and builds bulging muscles but is not oxygenating the body correctly – fresh air is still needed.

Stale recycled air is unhealthy and not doing your immune system a favour; nor is jogging in a haze of traffic fumes or running round the block in inner cities.

This can all add stress to the body, adding to a toxic body burden, which further reduces immunity.

Marathon runs can also be extremely taxing on the body; instead of gaining good immunity from exercise, you can lose it from the extreme stress the body is put through.

Intense exercise in extreme sport can cause lowered immunity, putting a person more at risk for infection and development of degenerative disorders.

Getting out into fresh air, joining hiking or walking groups and outdoor sports activities, will oxygenate and invigorate the body.

Do gentle to medium level sport, but if you are a determined extreme sport fanatic, then at least seek the advice of a reputable sports nutritionist, who can guide you through the type of diet you need and advise you on vital nutrient requirements to help your body systems recover.

## Irregular sleep pattern

Good immunity depends on a well-rested body. Getting to bed before midnight brings dividends. An ideal sleep pattern for keeping sleep hormones in balance, is to sleep from 11 p.m. – 7 a.m. The body responds well to routine.

Deep restorative sleep in stage 3, when cells are best regenerated, takes place in the first half of the night. Establishing a regular sleep pattern will also help your immune function. Supporting your biochemical body clock by having regular bedtime hours allows you to wake refreshed and ready for action.

Circadian rhythms control your wake/sleep patterns. We produce the sleep hormone melatonin when darkness sets in, so it is best to avoid bright lights before sleep, as this can disturb your natural body clock.

Switching off computers and electrical devices in the home can improve quality of sleep; this includes removing battery-driven watches from your arm.

## Traffic fumes and airborne chemicals

Toxins from inhaled fumes must be metabolised by the liver.

The detoxification pathways are supported by certain nutrients, in particular amino acids from protein.

You can't always avoid airborne pollutants but eating healthily can help you to detoxify these chemicals, as these ultimately make their way into the bloodstream and affect healthy brain and immune function.

## Food temperature

This is particularly important, as it can affect how well you digest your food. At certain temperatures, enzymes are destroyed – not only in food, but in your own production of digestive enzymes.

Throwing icy cold beer or piping hot spicy foods down your throat increases risk of digestive problems developing.

Do not fully boil the kettle, try to drink hot drinks at lower temperatures and eat sweet spices, instead of chili that has the potential to damage the gut lining.

## Environmental and recreational toxins

Smoking and drinking are social poisons. The human body adapts – to a degree – but risk of disease increases in the meantime. This is a personal decision, but if some facts were made clear to early smokers, perhaps they would think twice.

Smoking is a major promoter of free radical activity (explained in **Part Three**). Chain smoking causes irreversible cell damage.

Free radical damage can cause premature ageing. It oxidises cholesterol, increasing risk for heart disease, promotes cell damage and risk of cancer. High levels of free radicals in the body can seriously tax your immune system.

One puff of a cigarette contains between 1,000 and 4,000 different damaging chemicals for the human body, including carbon dioxide, hydrogen cyanide, ammonia, butane, propane, aldicarb, and methyl bromide.

Cigarette paper is soaked with carcinogenic chemicals, to reduce burning time.

Tobacco plants are sprayed regularly throughout the growing season with pesticides and herbicides – all these chemicals are highly toxic.

Do you want these poisons in your body? Is the 'fix' worth it?

## Oral care

Dental materials are not all good. Learn to query what is put into your mouth. Research the latest, biocompatible, safe, non-toxic materials used for fillings, repair work, implants or bridges.

Many standard cost-effective materials used by dentists contain fluorescents that give the 'glow' of natural teeth, or use other translucent composite materials that contain toxic additives: mercury, lead, uranium etc.

Enamel mottling and health problems can be caused by using sodium fluoride, which is best avoided (a by-product of aluminium smelting).

Calcium fluoride is the naturally occurring form of fluoride that should be used. The risk of ill health from absorbing other undesirable toxic chemicals in the dental industry, such as bisphenol A, solvents, methacrylate, formaldehyde, dibutyl phthalates, cadmium and dibenzoyl peroxide, is high.

There are many safe, non-leaching, biocompatible materials that can be sourced on request by friendly understanding dentists. Ceramics, Zirconium, silicon-based resins, calcium hydroxide.

These are the sort of material biological and holistic dentists use.

## HARMFUL CHEMICALS IN BODY-CARE PRODUCTS

### Aluminium:

A heavy metal that was, and still is, being used in anti-perspirants, antacid medication, antiseptic products and vaccines. Studies have linked this metal to Alzheimer's disease. All heavy metals that enter the human body will have a negative impact on immunity.

## Fluorocarbons:

Used in hair sprays as a propellant, it has been found to cause upper respiratory tract irritation.

## Formaldehyde:

Utilised as a disinfectant, fixative or preservative, this toxic chemical is found in many cosmetics. Used also in embalming processes. The human body cannot metabolise or excrete this chemical easily.

## Dioxin:

Potentially carcinogenic and used to bleach paper and produce containers for products, such as milk.

## Mineral oil:

A product made from crude oil (petroleum) and used as a lubricator in skin creams. It creates an oily film that stops the skin's normal respiration function and damages the immune barrier.

## Sodium Lauryl Sulphate:

A harsh detergent used as a cleaning agent and put into cosmetics. As a skin irritant, it is harmful when used long-term. It has been found to cause poor health in children and adults.

## Propylene Glycol:

A mineral oil used in hydraulic fluid and anti-freeze but also in cosmetics, skin and hair products. It is a harsh skin irritant.

**Alpha Hydroxy Acid:**

Used in skin care products as an exfoliator. This can damage skin cells and disturb the protective barrier, which is so important in immune response. Long term use can cause progressive changes in skin cells.

There are many other synthetic harmful chemicals used in the cosmetic and body care industry. Always read labels.

It is far healthier and safer to use herbal, chemical-free options. Not only are you buying for specific reasons to avoid artificial chemicals, but gain healthy nourishment for your body, with vital fatty acids, nutrients and plant pigments.

# PART TWO
# STRENGTHENING DEFENCES

## NUTRIENTS THAT MATTER

### Vitamin A

This valuable vitamin is a major antioxidant that works to keep cells healthy. It helps preserve integrity of your skin – maintaining the protective barrier that stops infectious from entering your body. It nourishes the mucosal lining of your respiratory, digestive and urogenital tracts.

The vitamin is also required for producing bacteria-fighting lysozymes (enzymes) in tears, saliva and sweat.

Vitamin A helps both the innate and adaptive immune systems, by helping production of your B and T cells which become active as infection strikes.

**The best foods for vitamin A content are dairy products, cod liver oil, apricots, broccoli, peas, and beta carotene – rich foods found in all orange coloured plants.**

**Beta carotene is converted in the body to active vitamin A.**

### B Vitamins

The full complex of water-soluble B vitamins – B1 (thiamine) B2 (riboflavin) B3 (niacin) B5 (pantothenic acid) B6 (pyridoxine)

B12 (cobalamin), folic acid and biotin are important for immune support.

They are required for antibody, B & T cell production, mucosal barrier maintenance, nervous system support, thymus and lymphatic function, and for improving phagocytosis: the process of destroying pathogens. Vitamin B3 is especially useful in helping to fight viral infections.

**Rich sources come from wholegrains, nuts, seeds, dairy products, eggs, beans, vegetables, fish, meat, poultry, mushrooms, greens, and wholegrain brown rice. Steaming foods with the lid on preserves B vitamin loss in steam.**

## Vitamin C

Vitamin C is probably the most important player in the nutrient field for fighting infection. It is called an essential nutrient because we cannot make vitamin C in our bodies: we must get it from our diet.

According to a recent placebo controlled trial in China, 80% less mortality was achieved in critically ill COVID – 19 patients given 24gm IV vitamin C daily. Refer to: https://www.vitaminc4covid.com. (Professor Peng, Zhongnan Hospital)

This is to be expected, as vitamin C in the ascorbic acid form has extremely powerful antioxidant, antimicrobial and anti-inflammatory properties.

The higher the dose, the stronger the effect. As a water-soluble vitamin, higher doses can be used safely, but it can also thin the blood so should not be taken by people on blood thinning medication.

Vitamin C is also a remarkable skin healer. Together with zinc it is required for production of new skin cells.

It acts specifically on the immune system by stimulating white blood cell production and increasing phagocytosis. The best way to nourish and saturate your body tissues for protection against any type of infection is with vitamin C.

An added benefit is its ability to reduce stress, beautify your skin structure with healthy collagen and improve digestive function.

Keeping guard throughout your body, vitamin C searches for toxic foreign material, viral, bacterial or fungal invaders – then forms a long tentacle, to reach out – envelop the invader and pull it into its own cell for final destruction.

Star wars at its best. The ammunition needed for this remarkable action is released inside the cell, in the form of enzymes and other substances – these strong agents rapidly destroy the invader.

**Vitamin C rich foods are mainly fresh fruits, tomatoes, salad and vegetables. Berries are extremely high in this valuable vitamin, the darker the better. Leaving the skin on potatoes reduces vitamin C loss in cooking.**

**Vitamin C works synergistically with bioflavonoids, the pigments in produce; by choosing fruits with intense colour, you will increase bioflavonoid intake. If supplementing, use a product containing both nutrients.**

## Vitamin D 'The Sunshine Vitamin'

This vitamin is required for many essential body functions. It also plays an important part in maintaining healthy immune function by enhancing phagocytosis.

When exposed to enough sunlight, sensibly throughout the year, without sun blocking cream, most people can maintain adequate vitamin D levels.

Recent research on immune function shows vitamin D to be more necessary than previously thought but a degree of caution should be applied. Some indigenous tribes in Africa, due to their genetic make-up, keep healthy, despite having naturally lower levels of vitamin D. The vitamin is also required for calcium absorption for keeping healthy bones.

Mega dosing for immune support may upset this delicate balance and is something to be aware of in the current trend of mass vitamin D dosing.

**Dietary sources rich in vitamin D are mainly from animal products: oily fish, sardines, salmon, herring, mackerel, egg yolk, red meat, liver and butter.**

## Vitamin E

As a major antioxidant, vitamin E helps protect your cells from damage. Oxidative damage is produced every day from normal metabolic function; it also occurs during the destruction process when immune cells kill infectious pathogens.

With its co-factor, selenium, these nutrients work hard to keep your cells healthy. Vitamin E also improves antibody production and helps phagocytosis: the process of destroying germs.

**Good dietary sources come from nuts, seeds, wholegrains – especially wheatgerm (preferably from ancient grains, not modern wheat), lima beans, sweet potatoes. and avocadoes.**

## Iron and Copper

Iron and copper are minerals that are required in tiny amounts for good health. but caution needs to be applied, as these can also be damaging for health when levels rise – usually resulting from inappropriate supplementation or taking synthetic hormones; that can cause disturbance in mineral balance.

These elements can also in certain instances increase risk of infection, so supplementation is unadvisable, unless deficiency or excess is shown in test procedures. and then, taken only under practitioner's guidance.

**Rich sources include wholegrains, nuts, seeds, cocoa powder, figs, apricots, beets, olives, leafy greens, mushrooms and shellfish.**

## Magnesium

Magnesium is required for many functions in the body. This mineral works together with calcium for muscle contraction and relaxation, is required for fat metabolism and digestive processes, for healthy heart function and nerve transmission.

A deficiency of this valuable mineral has been shown to slow immune response and increase stress.

**Good dietary sources include pumpkin seeds, beans, peas, brown rice, nuts, wholegrains, and dark green leafy vegetables.**

**Chlorophyll – the green colour in vegetables and green sea algae – contains high levels of magnesium.**

## Selenium

Selenium is an important antioxidant that keep your cells healthy. Together with vitamin E it is a part of an enzyme system that protects the integrity of your cell walls, inhibiting bacteria and viruses from entering your body.

It also helps antibody response and supports phagocytosis when infection threatens.

**Foods high in selenium include brazil nuts, cashews, tuna, poultry. Some countries in the world have extremely low selenium levels in the soil.**

**It may be best to supplement this vital nutrient in selenium deficient areas, together with vitamin E but never as selenium selenite. Selenium methionine is the form to take, at a maximum dose of 200mcg.**

**Most quality vitamin mineral formulas contain this level in the correct form for maximum absorption.**

## Zinc

Zinc is necessary for hundreds of enzyme reactions in the human body. It is required for dozens of biological processes, including insulin production for blood sugar control, adrenal function for stress management, reproductive health and the production of stomach acid to digest the protein in your food.

Zinc and vitamin B6 work synergistically together in most of these functions.

Your body cannot live without zinc; it is the one trace element that is easily reduced – together with vitamin C, magnesium and B vitamins – when you are under prolonged stress.

Zinc deficiency, in our stressful modern society, is linked to reduced immunity.

Other functions include antioxidant, B, T cell and thymus activity, which helps fight viral, fungal and bacterial infections.

There are two sides to consider when taking it as a supplement.

Zinc does promote T cell immunity however, taken in high dose 30-50mg supplement form, can also diminish phagocytosis and reduce immune cells: neutrophil and macrophage action, especially during bacterial or fungal infections. It is probably best to avoid supplementation when bacterial infection is diagnosed. However, zinc has shown good anti-microbial effects for fighting viral infections.

**Foods high in zinc include oysters, seafood, dairy, red meat, poultry, wholegrains, pumpkin, sesame, and sunflower seeds.**

## Essential fatty acids

Essential fats are necessary for good immunity, and for building healthy immune cells. Together with protein, fats are components of your cell walls.

Omega 3 supports healthy immune responses. Being part of every cell membrane, these oils act as a protective barrier against pathogens entering your body.

They are precursors to hormone-like molecules (prostaglandins) that have either pro-inflammatory or anti-inflammatory properties.

B vitamins, zinc and magnesium are needed to convert these fats, by enzyme action, into prostaglandins.

Eating the wrong fats can influence whether you develop inflammation or not. Trans fats are dangerous fats with a damaged molecular structure that can negatively affect your health.

Barbecued food and overheating to 'smoking level' of any untreated oil will produce trans fats. On the other hand, processed hydrogenated cooking oils that have been stabilised also contain trans fats, because the healthy molecular structure has been altered.

Trans fats are dangerous; they have been shown to be carcinogenic – having the ability to cause cell damage.

A healthy body requires all the omega fats but in the correct ratio.

Ideally 2:1 in favour of omega 3 which promotes anti-inflammatory action.

## Omega 3 rich foods:

Walnuts, linseeds, oily fish, seafood, non-hydrogenated plant oils.

## Omega 6 rich foods:

Sesame and sunflower seeds, green leafy vegetables, hazelnuts, blackcurrant seed oil, evening primrose, starflower (borage) and safflower oil, soybeans, eggs, avocado.

## SKIN AND IMMUNITY

Your skin is the biggest detoxifying organ. Skin cells are renewed every few weeks, so you can imagine how much raw material in the form of nutrients you need to keep it in good condition. Nutrients build new cells.

Your skin functions as a shield against environmental pollutants and microbial invaders. It helps you to absorb vitamin D from sunshine, regulates your body temperature, and helps detoxification of toxins entering your body in food.

It pays to look after it.

B vitamins, Vitamin A, C, E, zinc and essential fatty acids are all required for healthy skin.

A lack of essential fatty acids and B vitamins can cause eczema, dermatitis and other skin disorders.

**Adequate essential fatty acid intake can be achieved by eating a varied diet. Other essential fatty acids, from walnut oil, safflower, hemp or sunflower oil, should all be eaten unprocessed and cold pressed.**

**Olive oil can be used on low heat. Avocado or coconut oil can be used safely for cooking purposes that require higher temperatures.**

## NUTRIENT DEFICIENCY SIGNS:

### Vitamin A

Mouth ulcers, dry flaky skin, dry eye syndrome, cataracts, loose stools, acne, poor night vision, frequent colds, infections, dandruff

### Vitamin D

Joint pains and stiffness, poor immune function, hair loss, muscle cramps, tooth decay, excessive perspiration, low energy

### Vitamin E

Easy bruising, lack of sex drive, varicose veins, slow wound healing, dry skin, hormonal problems

## B Vitamins

Skin problems, bloodshot, gritty eyes, nerve disorders, stress, poor memory, poor hair condition, sensitive tongue, irritability, cracked lips, insomnia, headaches, sore muscles, nails, digestive problems, hormonal imbalance, lack of energy, hair loss, panic attacks

## Vitamin C

Poor skin healing, easy bruising, frequent infections, bleeding gums, loose teeth, low energy, stress, low immunity, digestive problems, hormonal imbalance

## Zinc

Poor skin healing, white striae skin scars on skin (in pregnancy), white marks on nails, poor sense of taste and smell, low sperm count, frequent infections, digestive problems, hormonal imbalance, acne, infertility, nausea, loss of appetite, eating disorders, mental disorders, panic attacks, poor immunity

## Magnesium

Digestive problems, muscle spasms, palpitations, nervous conditions, high blood pressure, cardiovascular disease, mental disorders

## Iron

Ridges on nails, sore tongue, pale skin, anaemia

## Copper

Hair and skin problems, loss of pigmentation, cardiovascular disorders, hormonal imbalance

## Selenium

Infertility, mental fog, poor focus, lowered immune function, fatigue, hair loss

Even mild deficiencies may reduce the effectiveness of your immune system. A balanced, varied diet will ensure you have all the dozens of nutrients that we require daily for good immune function, but other factors need attention – sleep, stress, dietary stressors.

## ACTION REQUIRED FOR IMPROVING IMMUNITY

### A well-balanced diet is the basis for good health and immunity

You may be the type of person that does pay attention to food choice and already eats healthily. In which case the section on nutritional supplementation and medicinal plants may be of more interest to you if you require immune boosting support.

For individuals who are on poor diets, it is well worth noting that organically grown, nutrient-rich produce can help protect you from disease. Building strong immune resistance, these foods can help you to both avoid and fight infection.

Simple measures; but in time, effective. This basic advice cannot be emphasised enough. Perhaps it is so simple that people feel it can't be that effective – but your body needs the correct fuel, and a pharmaceutical pill cannot provide that.

Building up strong resistance to disease is much easier than fighting infection once it has got a hold.

Experiment – make changes and note effects.

You can do a lot to reduce the stress of worrying about a virus heading your way – you can eat your way to better health – protect your cells from invasion. A weak, undernourished body is at more risk.

I not only promote these simple habits; I have experienced remarkable health benefits and reversal of disease in thousands of sick people, during my twenty-five years in practice – simply from changing bad habits and topping up with nutrients, even before specific treatment was applied.

Contrary to general opinion, this step is easy to implement. You will not be a 'killjoy' whilst out with friends, take it from me.

Times are changing. Exciting, colourful, healthy diets are slowly creeping into restaurant menus.

The trick is learning to source where the healthy restaurants are and introducing your sceptic friends to colourful nutritious food. Learning how to prepare tasty healthy dishes at home, where you can, can also impress guests.

The abundance of healthy organic food available just means one thing: there is no need for excuses, it is all out there for the taking; you just need to change your mind set.

A daily intake of rainbow coloured fresh produce, antioxidants, vitamins and minerals is your immune protection.

## Why eat organic food?

Organic farming bans the use of poisonous pesticides and herbicides; it is a sustainable system which produces healthy food by using crop rotation to replenish nutrients back into the soil to encourage nutritious crops.

Organic produce contains higher levels of vitamins and minerals compared to crops grown with intensive farming practices. This type of produce helps build healthy bodies and resilient immune systems.

Though more expensive than mass produced chemically grown food, organic food has been shown in numerous studies to support good health.

Studies testing the nutritional content of conventional produce versus biodynamic or organic food, has produced consistent results: higher nutrient levels in the latter.

Feeding our bodies with nutrient rich produce makes sense; avoiding pesticide and herbicide residues on our food also makes good sense.

Protecting our land and insect population with a sustainable system of farming, and renewing the soil with nutrients, may not be everyone's pet subject, but why not give a little back to nature?

A staggeringly high percentage of randomly checked, chemically grown supermarket produce has shown toxic residues way above the maximum safety levels. *The Living Earth* magazine.

The latest 2019 report called '*A Cocktail effect*' from *Pesticide Action Network* (PAN) UK, in collaboration with *The Soil Association*, identifies more than one third of all conventionally farmed fruit and vegetables in the UK as containing high levels of harmful pesticide residues.

The study revealed that 66% of water samples from river catchment areas containing over ten different pesticide residues, 67% of soil samples had multiple chemical residues, and 43% of bumble bees contained traces of seven different pesticides.

These figures are alarming and anyone reading this would be well advised to focus on organic food only.

The public are regularly exposed to harmful effects from toxic poisons.

Is there any wonder at the decline in public health?

Spraying toxins in the garden is poisonous to valuable insect life, and presents an added risk to humans, from inhalation or drift onto vegetable plots.

There are harmless alternatives that benefit plant, animal and insect kingdoms.

Why ingest poisons when there are alternatives?

Tons of pesticides are sprayed on agricultural land each year – repeat sprayings over the growing period, with hormone disrupting chemicals.

Add to this cosmetic chemical treatment processes your food is exposed to before it comes to market, and you can appreciate how easy it is to become overloaded with toxic chemicals that have no place or function in the human body.

## Food production

Gene-altered foods, flavour enhancers, artificial colours, preservatives and emulsifiers – the list goes on: over 8,000 chemicals are used today in the food industry.

Take note of how many times your chilled supermarket vegetables and fruit go off before you have a chance to eat them.

Chilling and gassing produce destroys vital enzymes. Without this practice, as an example – carrots will keep for a whole season when stored in the correct manner.

Unripe fruit is treated, to allow for home ripening. This in most cases, results in food that deteriorates quickly or is inedible.

This is the price we pay for stores packed full of goods flown in from around the world. Buying in local food markets is always best.

Fruit and vegetables kept at room temperature remain fresh for long periods of time.

In times of sickness, in puberty, pregnancy or old age, the human body requires higher levels of nutrients. Choosing to eat organic can take care of these extra nutritional requirements.

If you would like to feel well supported to ward off infection, then this is the route to go.

**Interestingly, on a German website called *Bionichtbio* (https:// bio-nichtbio.info), kirlian photography is used to assess enzyme activity (the sparks of life that nourish us), in organic and biodynamic produce.**

**The pictures from fruit and vegetables show amazing, beautiful healthy floral enzyme patterns.**

**In stark contrast, conventionally grown produce showed no enzyme patterns and inactive plant structure – the result of chemical damage. Hardly the type of food that enhances vitality and well-being – however well-balanced the meals are.**

Gaynor J Greber

## Toxins, Pollution and Food Production

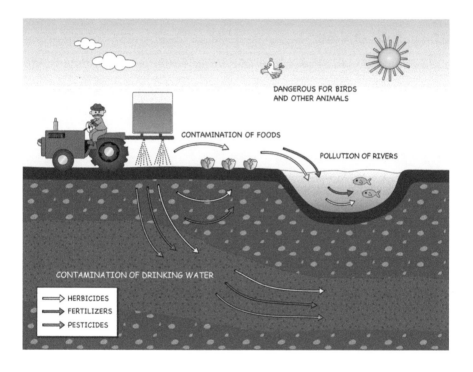

## Weight issues

## If you are struggling to maintain healthy weight, here are some useful facts.

Excess weight creates stress on body organs and tissues. Hospitalised patients who are overweight have been found to be less resistant to treatment and generally more prone to picking up infections.

On the *Obesity Action Group* website, it states that 'white adipose tissue slows down the immune response and has been shown to cause chronic low-grade inflammation'. Overweight people have also more difficulty fighting infections and are often left with more serious complications and ongoing health problems.

## Metabolic Syndrome

Studies reported in the *Science Daily* Journal, state that people with obesity and metabolic syndrome are at higher risk for picking up diseases and fighting viral infections.

Metabolic Syndrome occurs when individuals who are eating a high intake of carbohydrates develop a resistance to insulin. They are eating more carbohydrate than the body can metabolise. You could call this a pre-diabetic state. Another term used is Syndrome X or Insulin Resistance.

Every time you eat carbohydrates, which supply you with energy, your body produces the hormone insulin to put the glucose produced into cells for energy production.

The excess glucose gets stored in muscles and the liver. When your body runs out of glucose for energy, you have another hormone called glucagon, which converts the stored glucose back into cells for energy.

Insulin resistance causes premature aging, increases risk of cardiovascular disease and other degenerative diseases.

If the ratio between protein, fat and carbohydrate in your meals is imbalanced, and you are eating far too much carbohydrate – which produces sugar in the body – you can encourage the body to convert the excess sugar into fat.

Continue down this route, and the body stops responding effectively to insulin, because it has been struggling for so long to metabolise the sugar load.

People often insist they do not eat sugar! Just healthy foods. That may be true, but eating masses of bread, even wholegrain bread, is eating sugar! Fruit contains simple sugars; wholegrains contain complex sugars.

The result of digesting any carbohydrates, even vegetables – is sugar. Of course, add cane sugar to the mix and this really is overload. Not everyone eating a lot of bread will develop insulin resistance but some individuals, due to hormone imbalance, can be more at risk for this disorder.

## Fix the sugar fix

Constantly 'topping up' your blood sugar levels with a high intake of carbohydrates – can start a cascade of unhealthy changes in your blood fats if you develop Insulin Resistance. Triglycerides and cholesterol can increase, high density lipids (HDL) that keep fat from accumulating inside your cells can decrease, and low-density lipids (LDL) that help direct fat into cells can increase. In addition, blood glucose and insulin levels rise.

Imagine regularly eating more sugar than your body can handle – a diet high in refined processed carbohydrates, all your favourite fast foods which give a quick energy fix – processed white flour cereals, bread, cakes, biscuits, snack bars, white pasta, soft drinks, chocolate; and worse of all – sweets.

These goodies flood the body with what is called 'simple,' easily metabolised sugar: this hits the blood stream quickly and gives you your desired sugar fix.

You feel good for an hour or two – then you develop sugar cravings and off you go again – fulfilling a self-inflicted sugar addiction.

## Body fat and immunity

Body fat, or deep belly fat called visceral adipose tissue, often seen in men – secretes chemical substances called cytokines, that cause low level inflammation.

This inflammation can affect immune function, by reducing white blood cell activity. delaying immune responses and reducing function of the immune natural killer cells.

**According to recent reports in *The Guardian* newspaper, obesity has reached epidemic proportions in the UK.**

**The report states that one fifth of all adults are obese, and in the remaining population, half of the male population, and one third of all women are overweight.**

**If your diet is right for your body type – you will not be overweight.**

As already mentioned, you are biochemically unique, and so are your inherited nutritional requirements. Individuals each have specific needs for the kind of fuel that they can efficiently burn for energy. If you don't burn your food efficiently for your energy needs, it will be rapidly stored as fat.

Here, the plot gets tricky, because food can have virtually the opposite effect or influence in different people: foods that energise you, may cause fatigue and poor health in another individual.

This highlights the fact of just *how* individual we all are.

People also process foods and utilise nutrients at different rates. They may be a fast or slow metaboliser. How often have you wondered why a friend can eat something, that you find doesn't agree with you?

'One man's food can be another man's poison!'

## METABOLIC NUTRITION

### A simple measure to lose weight

By changing the ratio between carbohydrates, protein and fat in each meal, and eating complex (wholegrain) carbohydrates instead of simple (refined) carbohydrates, you can help burn off stored fat.

It is a simple procedure that does not involve calorie counting.

We need an approximate balance of these macro elements for good health, just visually having the largest portion on your plate as protein and the carbohydrate portion as non-starchy (containing less sugar) vegetables, will start the process of fat burning.

Eating only complex wholegrains in limited amount with plenty of protein (yoghurt, nuts seeds) and some fresh fruit at breakfast is a healthy plan. Alternatively, an egg pancake made with a protein rich grain taken with fresh fruit, nuts and seeds.

By reducing the carbohydrate content of meals, raised blood insulin, glucose and imbalanced lipid levels will normalise.

When you eat protein and fat your body does not produce insulin. Insulin promotes fat storage. So here we have a simple solution: eating more protein and fat can help burn off stored fat. Avoid snacking when you make these changes.

In good health, these are the approximate ratios you should be heading for:

55% carbohydrate from fresh fruit, vegetables, salad and wholegrains. (grains should be the smallest portion).

20% fat from nuts, seeds, plant foods, and oily fish. 10% from animal fat.

15% protein from fish, meat, eggs, dairy.

Specific foods can help you burn off fat more efficiently. Called the thermogenic effect these foods increase your metabolic rate, produce heat and increase metabolism. This can be greatly beneficial for weight loss.

**Green Tea, Apple Cider Vinegar, Mustard, Cinnamon, Tumeric, Garlic, Ginger, Paprika, Peppers, Bitter Oranges, Spices.**

## SUMMARY

- **Reduce carbohydrates and replace these calories with increased protein and healthy fat**
- **Drink plenty of plain water**
- **Avoid all added sugar, processed white flour products, alcohol and soft drinks**
- **Eat all carbohydrates, in a complex form: wholefood and unprocessed**

These are digested at a slower rate. They also contain fibre, which balances blood sugar and keeps the bowels healthy.

Digested over a period of hours, rather than a quick fix sugar rush, glucose is evenly distributed for energy needs throughout the day: stopping sugar cravings.

### Eat fat to burn fat

Fat gets metabolised at half the rate of carbohydrates. Heavier foods such as protein and fat, slow down metabolic function, and stabilise blood sugar. By calming the nerves – sugar cravings disappear.

Focus on increasing healthy polyunsaturated fats, (not animal fat) – avocadoes, olives, coconut, nuts and seeds and oily fish – to replace the carbohydrates you are reducing.

**Protein, together with fat, is required to build healthy immune cells.**

Eating light protein, dairy, eggs, lamb, poultry, seafood and fish in a ratio of 2:1 protein to carbohydrate will not only help the fat burning process but help supply you with immune support.

Using ancient grain (old spelt varieties, or Urdinkel, if you live on the continent) increases the protein content of your wholegrain carbohydrate meal portion. Rich in minerals and trace elements, it is well balanced from a nutritional point of view – containing on average 15% protein.

It should not contain any modern hybridized wheat, which is unhealthy, contributes to weight gain, and is mostly indigestible.

Digestive problems can often be cleared up purely by avoiding wheat. Modern wheat has been bred to be short and stocky and does not resemble old tall floppy wheat species plus the fact that the nutritional content of hybridized wheat is extremely low in comparison to ancient varieties of grains.

## Be a diet detective

The average western diet and lifestyle is geared towards acid forming foods. When food is digested, depending on what food it is, it leaves either an *acid ash* or an *alkaline ash* in the cells.

Digestive enzymes function within a slightly alkaline medium. This finely tuned balance can be disturbed by eating a highly acid-forming diet (alcohol, sugar, tea, and coffee), which often contributes to digestive problems.

Fruit and vegetables are your best alkaline foods – another reason to eat ample helpings daily. Wholegrains, fruit and vegetables, seeds, and nuts, all contain alkaline minerals: magnesium, calcium, sodium, potassium and zinc. The body uses alkaline minerals to calm the automatic nervous system. When you are stressed and uptight, the body becomes overly acidic. Acidity increases inflammation.

You can become mineral deficient when your body robs calcium out of bones and teeth, to help reduce body acidity – the result of you enjoying your acidic causing treats.

Any positive change made in diet and lifestyle is a step in the right direction. If you are prone to picking up infections, and have an unhealthy lifestyle, you need to give it some serious thought.

How far you wish to go in utilising the advice in this book is an individual choice.

Some experimentation to get the right balance between socialising and health would be a good idea.

Your body and feeling of well-being are the best judge if you have got it right.

## Reduce stress

During stress, the body releases a flood of stress hormones: adrenalin and cortisol – your blood pressure rises, your heart beat quickens, your body muscles tighten, and your brain gets into action for 'fight and flight'.

Identifying the cause of your stress and taking action to minimise it is the first action to take if you are under pressure and not coping well.

Physiological, psychological and emotional stress can all be interpreted by your body as stress.

This may be a poor diet high in stimulants, lack of sleep, demanding job, hectic lifestyle, blood sugar imbalance or intensive sports training. The effect is the same – adrenal stress. When your body is in stress mode it does not digest or absorb food well, so this can impact your nutrient balance and ultimately your immune system.

## Some basic steps you can take for stress reduction

Do not skip meals. Avoid stimulants – sugar, tea, coffee, cocoa or chocolate, sugared fizzy drinks and processed foods – you are probably already on a 'high', you do not want to be hyped up further.

Make certain your diet is well balanced with protein, fat and carbohydrate at each meal.

The net effect of eating regular well-balanced meals, is that these calories will help maintain good blood sugar levels, improve mood, reduce irritability, provide adequate energy and decrease fatigue.

If protein and fat are increased, there will be a calming effect.

Don't reach for sugar in any form when you are under stress; you are further undermining the body with simple carbohydrates that will rev you up again. Eat a protein snack instead, such as cheese and apple, to help reduce stress and make you feel relaxed.

Make certain you are not de-hydrated; a glass of water may not feel enticing but taken as a warm drink diluted with some protein in the form of nut or soya milk can be soothing.

Eat sugar-free snacks – dried fruit, always combined with nuts or seeds or other protein – to balance the concentrated carbohydrate. Or nuts, seeds, cheese, wholegrain crackers and fresh fruit, olives, avocado and carrot or celery sticks.

The B vitamins, zinc, calcium, potassium, magnesium, vitamin E and selenium in these foods further support the adrenal glands together with vitamin C, found in fruit and vegetables.

Eat plenty of protein at each meal, and healthy cold-pressed fats and oils, dark green vegetables that contain magnesium which helps calm the nervous system.

Eat fermented foods to nourish the gut bacteria. Eat in a relaxed calm environment, chew well and do not rush meals.

Feeling positive and in a good frame of mind is essential for improving immunity. Keeping both body and mind in an upbeat state will have a beneficial knock-on effect for the immune system.

Think holistically. Ask yourself whether all your body systems are well supplied with nutrients from your diet. Think whether you have adequate 'me' time for relaxation, personal enjoyment, hobbies or sport. Whether you have a good daily dose of sunshine, fresh air and exercise?

If you have anger to deal with, taking part in meditation may help. Deciding to make decisions to nourish yourself correctly and reap the benefit of a healthy body, can also improve mental calm.

A lot of the world's problems will always be there, so it is better, if not directly involved, to take a step back for your own peace of mind, and look around your immediate space, to enjoy what you have.

# PART THREE
# NATURE'S PHARMACY

**Food not only provides calories to stop you feeling hungry; it provides nutrients called phytochemicals to help protect you from infection, reduce inflammation and fight disease. These phytochemicals are found in fresh fruit, vegetables and herbs – super foods which help provide natural protection against infection, and support for the immune system.**

## Phytochemicals

Substances in food called flavonoids can prevent germs from taking hold and spreading. Quercetin, a flavonoid found in onions, citrus fruit, dark greens, apples, buckwheat, and other foods, has been found to have anti-viral properties.

It attacks the genetic material in viruses, stopping them from multiplying. Sulforaphane, a phytochemical in cruciferous vegetables – kale, broccoli, cabbage and Brussel sprouts – helps liver detoxification processes, and supports healthy hormonal function.

Another phytochemical called Resveratrol found in dark grapes, peanuts and the cocoa bean, acts as an antioxidant, protecting cells from oxidative damage.

Anthocyanins, members of the bioflavonoid phytochemicals, found in red, purple, blue, black berries, red wine, vegetables, salad, and other foods, have been mentioned in folk medicine worldwide.

## What is a free radical?

These are damaging compounds produced naturally by the body during normal metabolism, such as breathing and the process of digestion. They are controlled and regulated by antioxidant action.

We have two main strong antioxidant systems in our body to do this job – superoxide dismutase (SOD) and glutathione peroxidase (GP). These enzymes are dependent on nutrients from diet. Therefore, eating a nutrient dense diet is most important in mopping up free radical damage.

Scientific studies have demonstrated potent healing benefits for a range of conditions – including cardiovascular disease and eye health.

As free radical scavengers and antioxidants, phytochemicals are invaluable in the role of body protection against cellular damage.

Eating burnt foods, breathing in exhaust fumes, being exposed to toxins and pollutants, dangerous levels of sunshine, strenuous exhausting exercise, eating hydrogenated processed cooking oils – all increase the body's load of free radicals.

## What is an antioxidant?

Antioxidants fight to keep cells healthy by disabling the free radicals. They do this important task by joining force with enzymes that act as neutralisers.

Antioxidants in Food
Keep Cells Healthy

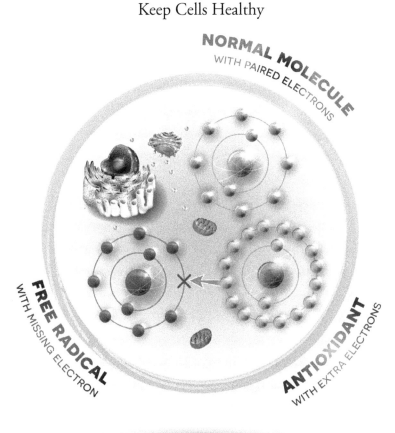

These important enzyme systems are dependent on vitamins and minerals, such as vitamin A, C, E, CoQ10, selenium, zinc, manganese, copper and iron – a range of nutrients that nature provides us with for protection from oxidative damage from free radicals.

This is our antioxidant defence army – nutrients and plant compounds that keep us healthy. The more mankind discovers, the more we can marvel how everything in nature has its place.

The body is constantly at risk of infection from harmful organisms in the environment, in addition to those that come into the body from food, but we have protective support from nature at hand.

You do not have to look far for natural treatment to boost immunity and fight disease.

## Antioxidant rainbow colours

Mangoes, pumpkin, carrots, yellow, red, orange peppers, all green leafy vegetables, root vegetables, citrus fruit, onions, garlic, ginger, berries, apricots, peaches and papaya, artichokes, tomatoes, spices and herbs offer a huge variety of disease fighting chemicals.

## The wider the variety, the better your support.

Eating a fresh, varied, colourful mix of antioxidant rich foods, spices and herbs is the best way to improve and boost immunity.

The stronger the defence, the better your state of health and resistance to disease.

Research studies throughout the world have indicated many benefits from the medicinal properties in plants. Herb and plant chemicals have been found to be effective in fighting infection and symptoms of ill health.

They can offer an alternative approach to pharmaceuticals for treating chronic disease as anti-inflammatory agents and pain killers.

## Healing properties in food and plants:

- cholesterol lowering, anticoagulant decongestants, expectorants
- anti-depressants, antibiotics, anti-inflammatories
- tranquillizers, antioxidants, analgesics
- insulin regulators, digestive aids, natural laxatives

## ANTIMICROBIAL POWER FROM MEDICINAL PLANTS

Herbs enhance our bodies' defence systems and strengthen immunity. Used therapeutically as supplements, they can bring immense benefit.

The active properties in herbs and plants vary considerably. Some can be taken quite safely according to the directions on the package, but for serious infections, people on medication or for specific health problems, it is recommended you consult a professional for advice on a specific herb's action, interaction with medication, and dosing procedure.

## Echinacea

Echinacea is a powerful well documented herb which supports immune function. It can be taken long-term to help prevent infection, perhaps in the winter months, or to help fight infection when you are sick.

It is also safe to use with children. Recent prescribing laws in Europe have changed the availability for children under twelve to be treated with this herb. It is my experience at half or quarter dose, to be most effective for younger children, this used to be the recommended dose.

Its action involves recognising pathogens and encouraging the immune system army to destruct. It strengthens and supports the immune system army of cells, rather like a General. Its action is not specific but rather broad-spectrum – helping in all areas of defence: a multi tasker.

When enhancing T cell action, it not only increases the body's ability to recognise pathogens, but also encourages the production of interferon (a signalling protein) which prevents viruses from replicating. The plant contains an active property in the roots, called chicoric acid, which helps increase phagocytosis.

One important role it plays, when taken during an infection, is to improve cell membrane defence, making cells less vulnerable to attack from invaders.

Echinacea has anti-inflammatory, anti-bacterial, antiviral and antiseptic properties.

Alfred Vogel, The Swiss Naturopath, mentions an incidence about echinacea in his book *The Nature Doctor*.

During a visit to the Amazon region, he was exposed to malaria by being bitten all over from mosquitos. His colleague succumbed to the disease, but Alfred Vogel had echinacea with him and took the tincture, forty drops morning and evening. He did not develop any symptoms and kept well.

Years later, a blood test showed he had had malaria at this time, but the infection had not produced symptoms.

He mentions a further incidence in his book, curing a bad case of blood poisoning from a scythe injury by chewing a whole echinacea plant and tying a swathe of crushed echinacea leaves around the wound. Rather old-fashioned methods, but nevertheless, it emphasises the potent healing power from this plant.

Scientific research confirms the efficacious effect of the echinacea plant, which contains a complex of active chemical substances. Its potency doesn't lie in using an extract form but in utilising the entire plant to retain the whole array of healing properties. It helps reinforce the body's own defence mechanisms, helping you to become more resistant to infection.

## Astragalus

Astragalus is an anti-microbial herb is used in Chinese medicine. Its usefulness lies in its ability to promote phagocytosis by increasing production of antibodies, interferon and T cells. It is a valuable tonic and toner for the immune system – improving energy and stamina, making it a good herb to take for chronic fatigue.

## Garlic

Garlic has been used as a medicinal plant by many cultures, over thousands of years. It contains significant amounts of vitamins and minerals, including selenium, so can provide additional nutritional support for the immune system.

Allicin is the main active ingredient in garlic. This has strong antibacterial, antiviral, antiparasitic and antifungal effects. These powerful effects work by stimulating immune function and increasing production of natural killer cells (NK) cells, a vital part of the body's defence army.

## Ginseng

Ginseng has been used for thousands of years in the Far East, as a general tonic for fatigue, stress and age-related complaints. It has been used to prevent disease and improve well-being by strengthening all body systems and improving resistance to infection.

Containing anti-viral properties, it boosts the body's immune defence system.

As an adaptogen, it can help the body withstand stress and has a toning effect on the glandular system, especially the thymus gland.

## Golden Seal

This herb is highly effective with a broad-spectrum effect – it activates macrophages in the immune system, is anti-inflammatory, anti-microbial, antiseptic, and acts as a general tonic by helping detoxification and bile flow. As an effective anti-germ agent, it has a wide influence throughout the body and can be used both topically and internally.

Topically it acts as an astringent, providing healing benefit to damaged skin; internally it helps keep a healthy mucosal lining in the lungs and gut.

## Pau D'arco

An herb used by the Amazonian Indians for centuries as an agent for wound healing, it has potent anti-viral, antibacterial, and anti-inflammatory properties.

As a pain-relieving anti-infective agent, it is remarkably effective in fighting infectious disease. For fungal health problems, it is particularly useful in reducing overgrowth.

## Nigella Sativa (NS)

These black cumin seeds from the Nigella Sativa plant are beneficial in many ways. They contain an active ingredient called Thymoquinone. The Egyptian species has the highest therapeutic medicinal activity. There are interesting reports of NS being used to treat hypertension.

These seeds have strong antioxidant, anti-microbial activity, are anti-inflammatory and antiseptic. Having analgesic effects, they can also be of further benefit for pain reduction.

## Boswellia

A tree that exerts many medicinal benefits – anti-inflammatory, immune enhancing, and anti-microbial. Frankincense is the oil extracted from this tree – used as an age-old remedy since biblical times.

Used topically, it is anti-bacterial, has antioxidant properties, and can help fight fungal overgrowth. Boswellia taken internally has analgesic, anti-inflammatory actions.

## Turmeric

Is a spice that has specific beneficial properties. Its active constituent, curcumin, can help fight inflammation during infection. It has a therapeutic role to play, in regulating and controlling production of inflammatory substances released by the immune system during defence function.

## Pine Bark

This extract from the bark of the French Maritime pine tree is a beneficial bioflavonoid that has strong antioxidant properties. It helps immune function by modulating antibody response and reducing production of inflammatory substances produced during an infection. *Pycnogenol* is the patented name available for purchase.

## Quercetin

This flavonoid found in many plants – buckwheat, red onions, fruits and seeds – is a phytochemical with unique biological properties; it can provide many health benefits for allergy treatment, cardiovascular health, muscular skeletal health problems. It has strong anti-inflammatory effects.

# Ginger

An all-round culinary and medicinal plant.

It has anti-spasmodic and anti-inflammatory actions and reduces fever by promoting perspiration. It can, at the right dose, also kill parasites and bacteria, by providing a disinfecting effect in the gut.

# Black Elderberry (Sambucus nigra)

Black elderberry contains active anti-viral substances.

The work of *Dr Madeleine Mumcuoglu* in Israel in 2006 highlighted ground breaking research, which identified the key active component in black elderberry that not only stopped viral invasion, but neutralised activity if some invaders had managed to reach the cells.

As viruses cannot reproduce themselves, the infection is then controlled and defeated.

A standardised patented elderberry extract called *Sambucol* was found to be effective against viral transmission.

A British Medical Research Institute associated with Queen Mary's College, University of London, announced in 2006 that *Sambucol* was at least 99% effective against the avian flu strains.

Just a further word about this useful berry. Do not eat it raw; it contains chemicals that detracts predators. It should be prepared by gentle cooking or bought in prepared form.

# Thuja

Is an herb that contains anti-viral properties. It is usually taken as a homeopathic remedy, under professional guidance of a Homeopath.

## Olive Leaf

Olive leaves have been used throughout history to support good health.

Medicinal properties in the olive leaf include antimicrobial and antiseptic activity. The leaf inhibits infection and reduces microbial and fungal growth.

The active components oleuropein and hydroxytyrosol inhibit pathogen invasion. Overall, they boost immune function and protect against infection.

## Medicinal Mushrooms

Medicinal mushrooms make up a large group of healing organisms.

Combinations of certain fermented medicinal mushrooms have extremely potent beneficial effects on the immune system.

There are thousands of mushroom species, many including Shiitake, Maitake and Reishi offer strong support for the immune system.

As anti-viral, anti-bacterial and anti-fungal foods, mushrooms enhance production of natural killer cells and increase macrophage activity by supplying powerful immune-modulating effects which help fight infection.

They specifically enhance innate immunity and have powerful immune boosting therapeutic properties.

Often used in natural cancer therapy, they have been found to help tumour regression.

## Artemisia annua

This is an extremely potent herb that helps fight infection. It has been shown to protect against malaria in the correct dose and is often more successful than Larium or other synthetic drugs in the fight against malarial disease.

Recognised as one of the most potent anti-microbial therapeutic herbs, many research studies are underway to test its full potential against viral infection.

The plant stimulates immune function, is anti-spasmodic and has anti-fungal properties.

## Berberis

Another very potent anti-microbial herb, berberine, the active component is particularly good for clearing up bacterial infections. It has an antioxidant, anti-inflammatory effect. Extremely effective in treating bacterial overgrowth and gut inflammation.

It protects the gut lining by acting as a powerful natural antibiotic, at the same time having a soothing healing effect.

It is effective also against fungal overgrowth, and is a strong activator of macrophage activity, helping to destroy bacteria, viruses, yeasts and tumour cells.

Berberine has shown anti-mucolytic effects, helping to clear mucus and phlegm from respiratory passageways. It stimulates bile and digestive enzyme production and increases blood flow to the spleen.

By all these measures, it can offer vital support for keeping intestinal health. Many chemicals contained in the dried bark have antiviral and anti-amoebic properties.

It is my personal favourite remedy, used for years in my nutritional clinical practice for treating gut disorders and never failing to bring relief.

## Cats Claw

The bark and root, popular in folk medicine, contains properties that have many immune stimulating effects. It is antioxidant and anti-inflammatory, and has a calming, healing effect on an inflamed gut.

Used in Peru to treat viral infections, it is recognized as a unique herbal therapy for gut related conditions.

## Citricidal from grapefruit seed

Grapefruit seed extract offers a broad range of antimicrobial effects. It treats fungal overgrowth and is powerful and effective in the control of bacteria and viruses. It can be used internally and topically.

## Oregano

This herb can be used to fight any opportunistic microbe. It contains Thymol and Carvacrol, extremely potent antimicrobial chemicals. Used internally in an essential oil concentrated extraction – it is so strong; it can mostly only be tolerated in small doses of 2-4 drops in a large glass of water. *Zane–Wild Oregano Oil.*

The oil can be used for both respiratory and gut infections.

Medicinal Herb - Berberis vulgaris

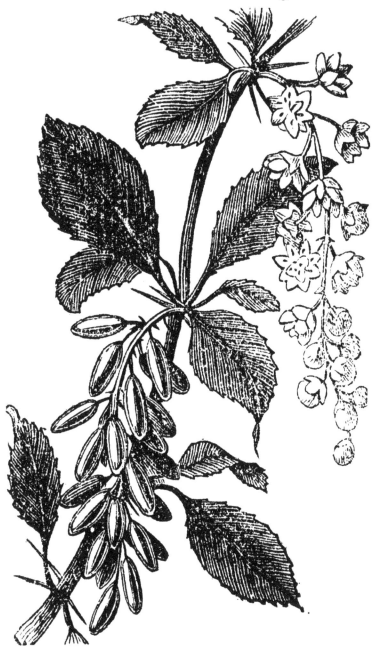

## Thyme

The herb Thyme also contains Thymol which has antibacterial properties that have been found to help fight infection. Only certain essential oils are safe to use internally, otherwise topical or culinary use of the herb is best.

## Hypericum (St John's Wort)

This plant contains Hypericin, an active compound that interferes with viral proliferation. It possesses antifungal and antibacterial properties. Caution should be applied when taking supplements as skin reactions to sunlight have been reported.

The herb can also react with certain drugs and hormone preparations. It would be best to seek professional advice if you are on medication.

# BOOSTING IMMUNITY WITH SUPER FOODS

## Chlorella and Spirulina

Algae plants are packed full of nutrients and plant chemicals. They are super concentrated whole foods that provide excellent sources of vitamins, minerals, trace elements and enzymes.

Containing high levels of complete protein, the nine amino acids that are essential for life, a range of essential fatty acids, and numerous plant chemicals that promote human health and boost immunity, these are true super foods.

The chlorophyll (the green pigment) is a rich source of magnesium, required for many body functions, a mineral that helps to reduce stress and anxiety. This green pigment is an excellent agent to help the body detoxify as it binds (chelates) heavy metals and other toxins, for excretion.

If used for detoxification purposes, professional monitoring is advised.

Algae can supplement nutrients that are mostly lacking in processed diets. They provide instant nourishment, long-lasting energy, and can be used as a general tonic for individuals who require extra nutrients: convalescents, young fussy eaters, teenagers, the elderly, and intense sport fanatics.

Both Chlorella and Spirulina are also rich in antioxidants, specifically beta carotene which supplies vitamin A at levels far higher than in carrots.

Used in smoothies, these foods can boost the health of body systems with concentrated goodness.

As we age, our immune function decreases, and the body's repair system begins to fade.

This, aside from poor dietary habits or faulty lifestyle, can make us more susceptible to disease.

We can't influence the process of aging, but we can ensure that we age healthily.

Chlorella has been found to stimulate the immune system by increasing macrophage and lymphocyte production. Studies have also shown that chlorella increases the body's resistance to viruses, helps fight free radical damage and keeps our liver functioning well.

## Honey

In its pure unadulterated form – not blended, or heat treated – honey offers numerous health-giving properties. It can be used as an antibiotic internally or topically as an antiseptic agent. It contains small amounts of B vitamins, vitamin C, calcium, iron, zinc, potassium, phosphorus, magnesium, selenium, chromium, manganese, enzymes, flavonoids and amino acids.

Used in moderation during infections, honey can disinfect, nourish and help increase antioxidant activity.

Bear in mind that the natural sugar content in honey is high and could provide fuel for bugs; this food is not recommended as a food source during ill health, rather a therapeutic medicinal treatment to be used prophylactically or during an infectious period.

## Propolis

Propolis has been shown to increase the action of phagocytes in destroying germs. Studies have shown some bacteria to be more sensitive to propolis than to synthetic antibiotics. Other studies have shown that propolis can kill fungal and bacterial infections.

Derived from the resin in bark, which bees collect to protect their colonies from bacterial and viral infection, propolis can provide a good defence against and during sickness. Taken during an infection, propolis, which contains bioflavonoids, can help control the number of invading micro-organisms and help stimulate the immune response.

It has anti-microbial, antioxidant, antiseptic and immune modulating properties.

## Royal Jelly

Bees secrete this substance from pollen to feed larvae and the queen bee. It contains many nutrients similar in composition to pollen, and numerous flavonoids that possess anti-viral, anti-inflammatory, anti-bacterial, antioxidant and disinfecting properties. Royal Jelly contains an acid which acts as a natural antibiotic, extremely useful to use against any infection.

## Pollen

This is a complete food containing most identified nutrients. It contains about 60% carbohydrate, 20% protein, 7% fat, 7% water, and the rest in the form of minerals or trace elements. The range of B vitamin content is high; vitamins C, D, E, K and carotenoids are present in small amounts. Pollen contains numerous other substances and enzymes that have health benefits for humans. It is a complete food that builds up cellular strength in all body systems.

Pollen can also increase resistance to infection and disease and improve energy and vigour.

Your body is a finely tuned engine that needs quality fuel to run well. As a tonic, when run down or under stress, or in times of need when infection threatens, we should look to the bees.

Optimum Nutrition means providing the body with as many extra nutrients and plant chemicals you can source – over and above a well-balanced diet. Differing food production methods means the nutritional value of each food varies.

By providing the body with levels of nutrients, in excess of the recommended Government guidelines – which, by the way, only indicates the levels required to avoid deficiency diseases, you can ensure adequate storage levels to maintain good health.

To keep fit and healthy, the human body requires optimal levels of nutrients, way above the recommended doses.

When the body is optimally nourished, you will have increased resistance to disease, resistance against infection and plentiful reserves stored in your cells.

## LOTIONS AND POTIONS

### Essential oils

Aromatics have been in use for millennia. The Greeks, Romans, Arabs, Persians and Indians all had their favourite aromatic potions and lotions and were very adept in distilling and mixing.

Ayurvedic medicine, from India, uses aromatic massage as a means of healing. Rose water for instance was prized for export all over Europe, the middle East and China. The active component is distilled from the plant and harvested at certain times when volatility is at its best.

Essential oils have potent anti-microbial properties and can rapidly be absorbed and reach the bloodstream. As the oil is in a small molecular size, it can easily penetrate your body tissues.

Inhalation can relieve stress, fight infection, harmonise mood, and balance hormones.

The fragrance from these concentrated essential oils can have a profound overall positive effect on health. They can soothe, reduce tension, stimulate the nervous system and improve concentration and mental awareness.

Various oil combinations alter brain waves to provide a heightened sense of wellbeing. Essential oils exert this influence via the *Limbic system* – the emotional part of the brain, which controls stress, hormones, breathing and your heart rate.

With a practitioner's expertise, certain combination of essential oils, appropriate to individual requirements, can be applied through massage.

Alternatively, you can make up your own anti-microbial or calming combinations by mixing your selection with a carrier oil and decanting into a small glass roller container bought from a chemist.

Apply this daily to the pulse points on your body for effective infection control, or use a relaxing combination rolled around the neck before bed, to calm the body and induce sleep.

By reducing the number of infectious bacteria entering your body, there is less chance of you getting sick.

Cleaning your face with an herbal face wash can quickly clear bacteria from nose, eyes, ears and sinuses, reducing your risk of picking up a bug.

There are wonderful anti-microbial sprays for body and face – handy to carry with you, if exposed to crowds and the threat of infection.

Organic lavender, patchouli or neroli sprays have a protective effect, and at the same time nourish and soothe your skin.

Spraying your personal room space will deliver good protection. There are many healing properties in essential oils but be sure to buy only organic and certificated oils. You do not want any contaminated products on your skin or in your lungs.

Airborne infections are caught from people sneezing and coughing in your vicinity. Carrying an anti-microbial herbal essential oil air spray will help counteract this risk by immediately disinfecting your space; you can also give a short spray on face masks.

Some oils have powerful antibiotic effects that can surpass the effects of antibiotics.

All essential oils have anti-microbial properties in varying degrees. If you are using them for extra support for fighting infection, you will need to research which oils are best suited to the type of infection you have. They offer protection from bacterial, viral, fungal infections and parasites. Useful also to apply with the common cold.

Some examples are: Neroli, Patchouli, Tea tree, Lemon, Juniper, Thyme, Cinnamon, Clove, Sandalwood, Marjoram, Oregano, Sage, Lavender, Rosemary Bergamot, Geranium, Myrrh, Melissa, Cedarwood, Wintergreen, Boswellia, and Myrtle

Essential oils contain numerous bioactive chemical compounds – including terpinine, pinene, carvacrol, linalool, limonine, thymol, terpenes and phenols, to name a few – that exert an antiseptic and germicidal effect.

They are often referred to as *Volatile oils.*

There are many oils too that can cause skin irritation, should be avoided in pregnancy and are simply not advisable for home use.

You should seek guidance from an Aromatherapist, if in doubt. They should also not be taken internally, unless otherwise stated on the instructions, or advised by a practitioner.

## ENZYME THERAPY

Apart from enzymes that digest food (protease, lipase and amylase) and metabolic enzymes that help keep our body functioning well, there are types of enzymes that help clear up infection and directly support our immune system during an infectious period.

They act as 'clearing out' agents – gobbling up pathogen residue, undigested food and generally cleaning up tissues, hoovering the debris that clogs up blood vessels, all the waste residue that must be eliminated out of the body.

Enzymes have many functions. We need digestive enzymes to break down our food. They are the 'spark plugs' of life.

Every biochemical reaction in the human body needs enzymes to function; from digestion to breathing, from fighting disease to controlling inflammation. The human body cannot exist without them.

As we age, our ability to produce and maintain adequate levels of enzymes that keep us fit and in good health declines.

This is a time in life when we especially need to increase intake of enzyme-rich foods in fresh fruit and vegetables. Enzymes in food only have a certain life span and are very fragile.

Our daily intake of food is mostly cooked, which destroys enzymes and nutrients; so ample portions of raw, enzyme rich foods from the plant kingdom, such as fruit and salad need to be eaten.

Long-term storage, supermarket lighting, transportation and intensive farming, can all destroy and reduce enzymes in food. Chilling or freezing food has the same effect.

## Serrapeptase – nature's gift

This enzyme originally originated from silkworms – an enzyme that the worm used to digest the cocoon surrounding it.

Today it is synthetically produced through fermentation of the micro-organism *Serratia E15*.

Serrapeptase has special features, digesting non-living tissue and acting as an anti-inflammatory agent.

It is called a proteolytic enzyme, because it can digest protein, and can help dissolve dead tissue.

These enzymes been found to be beneficial in clearing out blood clots, cysts, arterial plaque, and in the case of lung infections, clearing up mucus and catarrh.

By destroying the *Biofilm* – a protective barrier built by disease causing bacteria, – breaking down debris surrounding the walls of viruses, this enzyme can play an important part in helping to fight infectious diseases.

Proteolytic enzymes can be used to help fight microbial infection by dissolving microbes. These enzymes work systemically, passing through the blood stream to reach all body parts.

Some proteolytic enzyme combinations can break down pathogenic material, reduce inflammation and accelerate the body's natural healing power.

So here we have another beneficial treatment for the immune system.

Enzyme therapy has been shown to increase anti-viral activity in the immune system, by reducing inflammation, stimulating immune reactions, destroying and removing waste material, and increasing circulation of antibodies.

Nutrients are then encouraged to the site of infection to initiate healing.

There are many conditions that can be treated successfully with enzyme therapy.

## Dietary tips for Immune support:

- A daily organic fresh fruit salad – seasonal, local, rainbow coloured
- Sugar-free, wheat-free grains, dates, figs, mixed seeds and nuts (chia, linseed, hempseed, sunflower, pumpkin seeds, walnuts, almonds, cashews)

After waking from restful sleep, we need a light diet full of anabolic (energy-providing) nutrients – an easily digested meal that improves our immune function for the day.

Sprinkle spirulina, chlorella and bee pollen, add sugar-free live yoghurt, or quark and lemon juice, plus 100% organic fruit juice. Mix all to a creamy mixture, (This will oxidise and go brown if not made up fresh each morning).

Quark and whey products contain glutathione, a powerful antioxidant for immune health.

## Supplement tips for Immune support:

- Add protein and medicinal mushroom powder to a super food green powder smoothie drink such as *Garden of Life Perfect Food*, or similar. This adds extra nutritional support
- Take glutathione in reduced or liposomal form. Containing three sulphur-containing amino acids, it help protect immune cells. The body makes glutathione, but levels are reduced by poor nutrition, environmental toxins, aging and stress
- Take milk thistle to boost the body's natural production of glutathione

Take a quality high dose multi vitamin and mineral supplement daily, with high dose B vitamin complex (50mgs) and extra vitamin C (1-2 g), to protect against infection and support healthy immune function. (liposomal form)

This is an insurance policy against deficiency.

**Lifestyle tips for Immune support:**

- Drink plenty of plain water throughout the day
- Take fresh air and exercise daily
- Clear up digestive health problems
- Get enough sleep and eat well balanced meals

## USING NUTRIENTS AND HERBS FOR FIGHTING INFECTION

If you feel an infection is threatening, dose up slowly with the oral products listed below, have a warm diluted apple juice and sprinkle in a liberal amount of ginger powder.

Take a tepid to medium heat bath with essential oils. Roll an essential oil combination around the lymph glands and on the wrists.

Pop to bed and keep warm to sweat it out. Sleep heals; do not attempt to carry on regardless.

The combined remedies should, within a couple of hours, bring relief. As you feel your body responding, you can repeat dosing.

**If symptoms worsen, you should seek urgent medical opinion.**

Most multi nutrient supplements do not have sufficiently high levels of individual nutrients to fight infection when immunity is low.

Topping up with specific nutrients can power up your immune function:

- Continue with a high dose quality multi nutrient product
- Take 2g of Vitamin C every two hours, until bowel tolerance is reached – a state of tissue saturation that causes loose stools. Vitamin C can be taken on an empty stomach with water or with food. Reduce to 6g daily split in three doses once bowel tolerance has been achieved.
- As symptoms improve, reduce further to 3g daily, split over the day
- Add an herbal product that has a broad-spectrum effect. I recommend berberine during an active infection. Take the full recommended dose (not with food). As symptoms improve, reduce the dose. Always monitor tolerance
- During infection, artemisia, pau d'arco or golden seal can be added. As infection clears, reduce the dose. Take according to the instructions but monitor tolerance
- Add an extra medicinal mushroom supplement; formulas are rich in beta glucans and polysaccharides that help support immune function
- Add oregano oil (four drops in water daily)
- Take echinacea for immune support
- Add 1,000mg of L-Lysine – this is an amino acid with anti-viral activity; at the same time, avoid arginine rich foods

- Take extra zinc – up to 50mg daily. When infection clears, reduce this amount to 15-30mg daily

If you are diagnosed with a serious viral infection and are in hospital, I repeat, that recent studies have shown good recovery rates, using 24gm of vitamin C intravenously. Refer to page 50.

Vitamin C is water soluble, so is not toxic in high levels. It will just be excreted through the kidneys.

**People with kidney disease, blood clotting disorders, or who are on anti-coagulant medication should seek the advice of a medic before anticipating taking vitamin C.**

## DIETARY GUIDELINES TO FIGHT INFECTION

**Cook** with juniper berries, herbs, and anti-inflammatory spices, such as turmeric, paprika and curry powder. Drink onion soup to stop congestion. Make organic chicken bone broth to aid healing. Increase levels of vitamin A, by drinking carrot juice.

**Avoid** wheat (inflammatory promoting), shellfish (can have microbial contamination), dairy products (mucus promoting), stimulants – sugar, tea, coffee, alcohol, chocolate (arginine rich), fizzy drinks and processed foods.

**Increase** intake of fresh fruit and green leafy vegetables. Drink concentrated fermented vegetable juices (*Biotta*) – but not beetroot.

**Increase** protein intake at each meal. Light meats, fish, eggs. Protein is needed to fight infection.

**Eat** healthy fats – olive, avocado, coconut, walnut oils, seeds, nuts and oily fish.

**Drink** plenty of water throughout the day and last thing at night. Warm, diluted, fresh organic apple juice and herbal drinks. *Original Yogi Spice* Tea has antimicrobial effects; in fact, the whole range of loose Yogi Teas are excellent.

Try to avoid teabags – a modern invention that hides poor quality tea and taints the flavour with paper residue. even if unbleached.

If 100% organic fruit juice is taken, make certain it contains berries, dilute it with three quarters warm water and add a dose of black elderberry juice (*Sambucus*). Elderberry deactivates viruses. Lemon and honey or apple juice and ginger make soothing warm drinks.

**When** suffering from catarrh or mucus, it would be wise to add in proteolytic enzymes to help the body clear out debris.

**Avoid** heavy proteins such as red meat and pork – you do not want to overtax your digestive system.

It is vital you replenish and keep up the supply of supplements until you feel well again, and then reduce doses to maintenance level and start to take probiotics to boost gut immune function.

**For people on medication, refer to your health care provider if you are considering taking supplements. Herbal products can interact with medication and some nutritional supplements may not be appropriate to take with certain drugs.**

# YOUR PROTECTIVE TRAVEL KIT

When travelling in foreign parts, it is always wise to take some natural preventatives for protecting yourself, and for treating any infection you may pick up. Drugs are best used for serious symptoms – when they can be lifesaving.

Taking drugs for minor illness or for protection will suppress your immune system and hinder the body's natural healing power.

## ANTIMICROBIAL SUPPORT

- Olive leaf extract
- Egyptian Black Cumin seed
- Vitamin C
- Garlic
- Berberine
- Gentian root
- Goldenseal
- Artemisia annua
- Grapefruit seed
- Pau D'Arco
- Caprylic Acid
- Myrrh
- Oregano/Thyme
- Black Elderberry
- Echinacea
- Black Walnut hull or leaf

- Aloe Vera

## IMMUNE TONICS

- Bee Propolis and Pollen
- Organic protein powder
- Medicinal mushroom powder
- Super green/red plant antioxidant powders
- Probiotic powders
- Spirulina

## MICROBIAL CLEANSE

- Milk Thistle
- Split cell Chlorella

You will not need all these products, but it gives you choices and options depending on which countries you are visiting. Tropical locations will require stronger products.

I would suggest taking a quality multi vitamin/mineral supplement with the plant formulas. (*Viridian/Terranova*) My personal choice for effective antimicrobial support is echinacea, berberine and artemisia. (*Nutri Advanced/Invivo*), Bio Revive, Beta Immune with Bio Clear GI (*Invivo*).

Use insect repellent neem for enclosed spaces and other non-toxic antiseptic plant sprays for disinfecting surfaces.

## Comments on supplementation

It is important to remember to listen to your body. When taking supplements – more is not always best. The berberine and the artemisia should be taken at different times of the day and started at a lower dose to see how you tolerate the products. Although the berberine is best on an empty stomach, if you feel more comfortable you can take it with food.

Use some of these remedies, when anticipating being in crowded enclosed spaces, on transport, in contact with animals, local markets with unhygienic food displayed, or when you are near the company of individuals suffering with infection.

## A final word

Seek professional advice on specific supplement combinations and doses.

Prevention is always better than cure. It allows for peace of mind: your insurance policy against disease. It is a myth to expect protection from a super drug if you continue in body destructive habits.

Maintaining super immunity helps prevent the entry of damaging bugs and toxins into the body. Overseeing your own health can improve confidence and take away fear.

Building up resistance by using natural antibiotics from nature means you are working with your body, not against it.

You can fight infection and heal, secure in the knowledge that you are not causing harm to your body. The efficiency of your defence system is purely down to you, and the quality of your lifestyle and dietary choices. We can't buy health with a pill; it comes from within.

I hope some of the advice in this book helps you along this route.

**Functional Medicine optimises health in all body systems.**

# BIBLIOGRAPHY AND FURTHER READING:

Michael Murray ND, Joseph Pizzorno ND, *The Encyclopaedia of Natural Medicine*, Three Rivers Press, (1998)

Dr Anthony J Cichoke, *The Complete Book of Enzyme Therapy*, Avery, (1999)

Robert Redfern, *Serrapeptase – The Second Gift from Silkworms*, Naturally Healthy Publications, (2004)

Jane McWhirter, *The Practical Guide to Candida*, All Hallows Foundation, (1995)

Stephen Terrass, *Candida albicans – How Your Diet Can Help*, Thorsons, (1996)

Dr John McKenna, *Alternatives to Antibiotics*, Newleaf, (1996)

Dr Paul Clayton, *Health Defence*, Accelerated Learning Systems Ltd, (2001)

Jack Challem, Burton Berkson M.D., Melissa Diane Smith, *Syndrome X*, Wiley, (2000)

Stephen Terrass, *Stress*, (Nutritional Health Series), Thorsons, (1994)

Leon Chaitow, *Food Your Miracle Medicine*, Thorsons, (2001)

Leon Chaitow, *Natural Alternatives to Antibiotics*, Thorsons, (2001)

Alfred Vogel, *The Nature Doctor*, Mainstream Publishing, (2003)

Thomas Bertram, *Encyclopaedia of Herbal Medicine*, Grace Publishers, (1995)

William L Wolcott, *The Metabolic Typing Diet*, Doubleday, (2000)

Geoffrey Cannon, *Superbug*, Virgin, (1995)

Robert Tisserand, *Aromatherapy for Everyone*, (1990)

Michael A Weiner, *Maximum Immunity*, Gateway Books, (1989)

Gaynor J Greber, *Chronic Digestive Disorders – Regaining Health with the Functional Medicine Approach*, Matador, (2018)

Lynne Mc Taggart, *The Vaccination Bible*, What Doctors Don't Tell You Publication (1997)

Stephanie Cave with Deborah Mitchell, *What Your Doctor May Not Tell You About Children's Vaccinations*, Wellness Central, (2010)

Lynne Mc Taggart, *What Doctors Don't Tell You – The Truth About the Dangers of Modern Medicine*, Harper Collins, (1996)

Dr Jonathon Brostoff and Linda Gamlin, *The Complete Guide to Food Allergy and Intolerance*, Bloomsbury, (1992)

Dr Keith Mumby, *The Complete Guide to Food Allergies and Environmental Illness*, Thorsons, (1993)

'What Doctors Don't Tell You,' *The Environment Handbook,* (1997)

Viera Scheibner, *Vaccination*, (1993)

Hal A Huggins, DDS. Thomas E Levy, MD., *Uniformed Consent – The Hidden Dangers in Dental Care*, Hampton Roads Publishing Co, (1999)

Leon Chaitow and Natasha Trenev, *Probiotics*, Harper Collins, (1990)

Ramiel Nagel, *Cure Tooth Decay*, Golden Child Publishing, (2011)

Dr Nigel Plummer, *The Lactic Acid Bacteria – Their Role in Human Health,* Biomed Publications, (1992)

Hasnain Walji, *Bee Health*, Thorsons, (1996)

Richard Passwater, *Trace Elements, Hair Analysis and Nutrition*, Keats Publishing, (1993)

Leslie Fisher, *The Clinical Science of Mineral Therapy*, The Maurice Blackmore Research Foundation, (1993)

Dr Lawrence D Wilson, L.D. Wilson, *Nutritional Balancing and Hair Mineral Analysis,* L. D. Wilson Consultants, Inc, (1998)

William A R Thomson MD., *Healing Plants – A Modern Herbal.* Macmillan London Ltd, (1980)

Andrew Chevallier, *The Encyclopaedia of Medicinal Plants,* Dorling Kindersley, (1997)

Bryan Hubbard, *Secrets of the Drug Industry,* What Doctors Don't Tell You Publication, (2002)

David Hoffmann, *Holistic Herbal,* Element Books, (1996)

Mathew Walker, *Why We Sleep,* Penguin Books, (2017)

Lynne McTaggart, *The WDDTY Dental Handbook. A comprehensive guide to the dangers of fillings, fluoride and other dental practices,* The Wallace Press, (2000)

# RESOURCES

## LABORATORY TESTING

The following laboratories provide testing procedures that are only available through professional health-care providers. Tests that are sourced directly via the internet should be interpreted by a registered practitioner.

Usually laboratories can offer information on how to find a practitioner in your area.

Invivo Clinical Ltd.
The Coach House, 3 Lewiston Mill,
Toadsmoor Road,
Stroud, GL5 2TE
+44(0)333 241 2997
www.invivoclinical.co.uk.

Regenerus Laboratories Ltd.
Aero 14, Redhill Aerodrome,
Kings Mill Lane, Redhill RH1 5JY.
+44 (0)203 750 0780
www.regenerus.labs.com

Genova Diagnostics.
46-50 Coombe Road,
New Malden. KT3 4QF.
+44 (0)208 336 7750
www.gdx.net

Biolab Medical Unit.
The Stone House,
9 Weymouth Street,
London W1W 6DB
+44 (0)207 636 5959
www.biolab.co.uk

To find a Functional Medicine practitioner–www.functionalmedicine.org/practitioner The Institute for Functional Medicine.

To find a Nutritional Therapist – www.bant.org.uk The British Association for Applied Nutrition and Nutritional Therapy.

Products can be sourced with practitioner prescription at www.naturaldispensary.co.uk

Lightning Source UK Ltd.
Milton Keynes UK
UKHW020804130122
397069UK00004B/31